5 INGREDIENT STAGE 3 KIDNEY DISEASE DIET COOK BOOK

FOR SENIORS

60-DAY MEAL PLAN

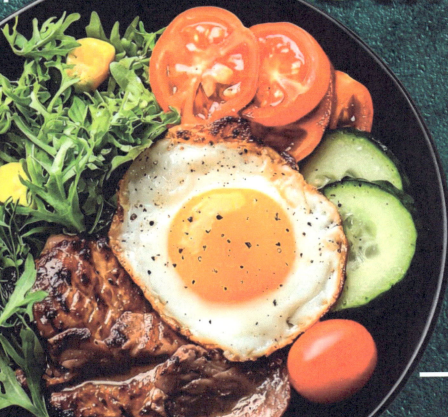

DIETITIAN APPROVED

FULL COLOR

MARIANNE GREENE

About Author

"Most kidney-friendly cookbooks I've seen are either way too complicated or just plain boring, which makes it hard for my patients to stick with them. This book breaks that mold completely. The focus on super simple shopping with ingredients that are easy to find, plus having only 5 ingredients or less per recipe, means my patients can actually enjoy cooking and eating healthy. I also really appreciate how the nutrition info is backed by USDA data — it gives me confidence to recommend it without worrying about accuracy."

— Randy M., Registered Dietitian (RDN)

"This is a great resource for patients with earlier stages of CKD. Easy to understand, with simple and delicious recipes. Definitely a great addition to your medical team recommendations to help you manage your CKD. I've been a renal dietitian for over 30 years, I can tell you it is important to balance your meals with all the different nutrients there are. The recipes have the amounts of important nutrients for your own balancing. Enjoy life with good food."

— Matilde Ladnier, U.S. Renal Dietitian (RDN), Member of National Kidney Foundation (NKF) - Council of Renal Nutrition (CRN)

"Cooking for my elderly dad is a challenge, but this book makes it easy with simple, step-by-step recipes that suit both American and European tastes. The meals are kidney-friendly and soft, perfect for seniors who don't want dialysis. Plus, everything takes under 30 minutes, which fits my busy schedule."

— Emily R., Family Caregiver

"My mom has always struggled with eating foods that are tough or crunchy, especially with her kidney issues. This cookbook is perfect because all the meals are soft, easy to chew, and made with real food proteins like eggs, chicken, and beans. The meals also hit the right calorie and protein levels to help her stay strong without overwhelming her with complicated dishes. The 60-day meal plan is a fantastic bonus — it keeps her eating balanced and gives me peace of mind."

— Linda K., Daughter and Caretaker of Senior Mom

"I'm 67 and was diagnosed with Stage 4 kidney disease with low eGFR. My doctor said dialysis was inevitable, but by following Marianne Greene's diet from this book, I've managed to keep my kidneys going strong much longer than expected. The detailed nutrition facts, especially the focus on low oxalates and controlled sodium, potassium, and phosphorus, helped me make safe food choices. The recipes are delicious and easy to prepare, which made sticking to the diet much easier."

— David G., 67, Stage 4 CKD Patient

Disclaimer and Legal Notice

Table of Contents

Table of Contents

Table of Contents

Table of Contents

Table of Contents

DRESSINGS TO ENRICH . .88

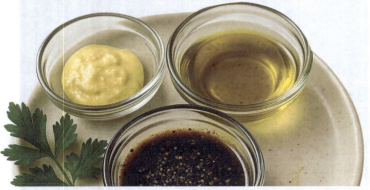

CONTINUE THE JOURNEY 90

RESOURCES 92

Grab your FREE Kidney-Safe Power Tools

◊ A game-changing Dining Out Cheat Sheet with smart swaps to order anywhere, red-flag items to avoid, and simple questions to ask your server.

◊ A CKD do-it-yourself Weekly Meal Planner to stay on track

◊ A Kidney-Friendly Grocery List for Smart Shopping

◊ Get your Detailed 60 day meal plan which shows nutrition sums. The Basic mealplan is included in the book already.

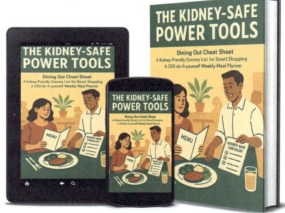

Scan this QR code to Claim your free gifts:

Authors Note

Hi, my name is Marianne Greene.

When my husband was diagnosed with stage 3 kidney disease, I already had over 17 years of experience working as a senior caregiver in assisted living homes. This gave me a deep understanding of the challenges seniors face—especially when it comes to eating well with kidney issues.

Over the years, I've helped countless people with chronic kidney disease, starting with the seniors I cared for and cooked meals for every day. I then supported my own family through kidney health challenges and expanded my reach to others facing similar struggles. Through my books, thousands of readers have found practical, kidney-friendly recipes that fit their lives.

One story I always love to share is about Mrs. Thompson, a retired teacher in her late 60s, with stage 4 CKD and a 22% eGFR.

On top of that, she was managing diabetes and arthritis, making meal prep physically challenging and time-consuming. Despite these setbacks, by following the simple, easy-to-follow recipes and meal plans I created, she was able to stabilize her kidney function and regain her energy—all without feeling overwhelmed or sacrificing flavor. If she can prepare these meals and avoid dialysis, I know you can too.

Why I Wrote This Book

After my husband's diagnosis, friends, family, and even old clients began asking: "Marianne, what are you making him? Can you share your recipes? Can you help us, too?" Dozens of requests later, I realized there was a huge gap between what people should eat and what was realistic to prepare day after day—especially for seniors or anyone juggling other health challenges, like arthritis, diabetes, or low energy.

My mission is simple: to make kidney-friendly eating accessible, enjoyable, and effective for everyone—no matter their lifestyle or background.

The CKD Stage 3 Challenge

Let's be real. Living with stage 3 kidney disease is tough, and most resources make it even tougher:

◊ **Confusing guidelines:** Potassium is bad—but sometimes it's good? Is phosphorus hiding in your bread? Is protein a friend or foe? It's exhausting.

◊ **Bland, boring food:** You see recipes for "boiled chicken and steamed cauliflower" and want to scream.

◊ **Complicated meal plans:** Six meals a day, specialty powders, expensive ingredients—who has the time, energy, or money for that?

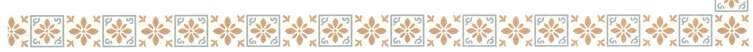

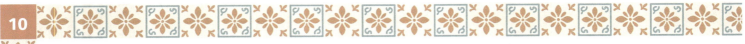

- **Physical challenges:** Maybe your hands or joints ache, or standing to cook is hard.
- **Emotional burnout:** You're tired of being told what you "can't" have. You just want a meal that feels normal.

Most "kidney-friendly" cookbooks are written by people who don't cook for someone with CKD. They're filled with complicated instructions, long lists of complicated foods, or bland recipes you'll never want to eat.

What This Book Is (and Isn't)

Let's be honest: This is a guideline, not a rulebook. I'm a caregiver who's walked this road and teamed up with two registered dietitians to get everything right.

Matilde Ladnier, one of the registered dietitians who reviewed this book and helped make it accurate is also available for consultations, you will find the link to contact RDN Matilde Ladnier at the end of this book in the "resource" section.

This book is not a replacement for your medical team. It's not a "miracle cure." It's a practical, supportive guide built by real people, for real life. Use it as a tool, alongside your doctor, your dietitian, your loved ones, and your own wisdom.

How is this Book Different

Most "kidney-friendly" cookbooks are way too complicated, boring, or just not made for real life. We made this one for you, to make eating healthy simple—and honestly, a little fun.

Here's what makes it different:

- **Reviewed by Dietitians:** Every recipe and meal plan has been carefully reviewed by a registered professional dietitian to ensure safety and nutritional balance.
- **Thousands of Satisfied Readers and CKD Warriors:** Our cookbook is trusted by thousands living with chronic kidney disease, helping them eat well and feel better.
- **The FIRST Book with a Meal Plan That Satisfies All Your Daily Macro Targets:** Unlike other books that leave you low on protein or calories, our meal plan hits every target to keep you strong and healthy. Not only we hit your Macros but in our meal plan you see the nutritional data for EACH meal and the TOTAL for each day.
- **Only 3 Meals a Day:** We know seniors don't want complicated 6-course days, so we kept it simple—high protein and calorie to keep everyone healthy and strong. We also include plenty of simple snacks and desserts. Plus, we leave room for calories, potassium, phosphorus, and sodium for each meal and day, as clear as it gets.
- **Soft Textures and Easy to Eat:** No tough to chew stuff. The meals are soft and senior-friendly (great if your teeth or jaw need a break).
- **Quick & Easy with Minimal Equipment:** Every recipe takes 30 minutes or less, with barely any equipment. Clean-up is a breeze. Perfect for busy people.

◊ **Overlapping Ingredients and Widely Available:** All the ingredients are widely available and easy to find at any big grocery store. You'll use the same overlapping ingredients in lots of recipes, so your shopping list is short

◊ **5 Ingredients or Less per Recipe:** Every meal has 5 main ingredients or fewer. No crazy long lists or complicated steps.

◊ **100+ Recipes and Lots of Flavor:** We change up the cooking styles and seasonings so you never get bored—think: egg salad, omelets, and poached eggs with salmon. Totally different flavors and textures.

◊ **60-Day Meal Plan:** No guesswork here, just straightforward, practical meal plans to keep you on track.

◊ **Nutrition You Can Trust:** We double-checked all the nutrition facts using official USDA data. (Note: They might change a little depending on the brands you pick, but it's about as close as you can get.)

◊ **Step-by-Step, In Order:** We list ingredients in the order you'll use them, so you don't get lost.

◊ **Oxalates Counted:** We included oxalate info (when it exists) to help you avoid kidney stones.

◊ **Healthy Energy:** We add olive oil for healthy fats and energy—but you can use less if you want fewer calories.

◊ **No Weird Abbreviations:** We only use "tbsp" for tablespoons. Or EVOO for extra virgin olive oil. Easy.

◊ **Real Food Only:** You get protein from real foods like eggs, chicken, and beans. No fake powders.

◊ **Fun Twists:** Want to try something new? Each recipe gives you a creative twist to play with.

◊ **Full Color with Pictures and Graphics:** Beautiful, full-color pages with pictures and easy-to-read graphics make following the book a breeze.

◊ **Aesthetically Designed to NOT Tire Your Eye:** Easy on the eyes, whether you prefer paperback or hardback.

◊ **Detailed Recipe Info:** Each recipe includes servings, prep time, cook time, protein, phosphorus, sodium, and potassium visual markers for quick reference, plus full nutritional info such as calories, carbs, and proteins.

We made every recipe to hit these health goals:

◊ **About 500 calories**

◊ **Low sodium (≤400mg)**

◊ **Low-to-moderate potassium (≤400mg)**

◊ **Low phosphorus (≤300mg)**

◊ **Good protein (15–20g)**

◊ **Low oxalates (≤50mg)**

How to use the book and NOT

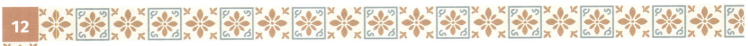

perfectionism

I want to say this as clearly as possible: You don't have to read this book from cover to cover. Start wherever you want. Flip straight to the recipes, browse the quick tips, read the background info—whatever works for you.

If you're tired, skip to a meal plan and follow it for a few days. If you're curious, dive into the nutrition guides and learn about what's really happening in your body. If you want to adapt a recipe, go for it! Swap the protein, change the herbs, tweak the texture. The goal isn't perfection—it's progress and pleasure.

Every recipe here is adaptable. If your doctor or dietitian gives you advice that conflicts with this book, always follow their lead. Bring them the recipes, share the meal plans. This is a tool to help you, not a rigid set of rules to make you miserable.

You're allowed to skip what doesn't fit, change what you need, and make it your own. Share this book with your family, friends, or care team. The more support you have, the easier and less lonely this journey will feel.

Final Words

Thank you for trusting me and letting these recipes into your kitchen.

Yes, better lab numbers matter. But what really counts is how you feel: more energy, less worry, real meals you look forward to, and days that feel normal again.

That's what we're after.

From my kitchen to yours.

With love,

MARIANNE GREENE

p.S.

If the pictures look great, it's because they were made in a kitchen studio, with great lighting and high tech cameras, don't get discouraged if yours don't look like them. They'll be just as tasty.

Join Our Private Facebook Group!

Living with CKD can feel isolating and overwhelming, especially when it comes to diet and lifestyle changes. In this group, you're not alone. You'll gain support from a community that truly understands what you're facing, get answers to your questions, and feel empowered with encouragement and resources tailored to your needs. Just search

"Kidney Disease Warriors: Stage 3 & 4 CKD Diet, Recipes and Community"

The group is on Facebook—we can't wait to welcome you.

Or Scan this and request to join our group <3

FAQs - 60-day meal plan

Q: Why are there no snacks or desserts in the daily plan?

We kept the plan simple and flexible by focusing on three main meals. You are encouraged to choose 1-2 recipes from the separate Snack & Dessert Section each day based on your personal hunger and calorie goals. We aim to hit 1500 calories with just the basic 3 meals. With 1-2 snacks of your choice, you are at 2000kcal.

Our recipes are low on Phosphorus, Sodium and Potassium, so you can double up if you need to. You can get the detailed plan with all nutritions for the meal plan listed with the QR code. The book contains the simple version with page numbers.

Q: I'm still hungry or I'm an active senior. Can I eat more?

Yes, absolutely. The plan is a baseline. If you need more calories, you can safely double the portions of any breakfast, lunch, or dinner as needed. Please use the provided nutrition facts to ensure your increased intake aligns with your doctor's overall guidance.

Q: What if I miss a day or have a "bad" meal?

That's normal. One meal won't undo your progress. Just start fresh at the next meal. If you find yourself slipping often, plan meals ahead or keep healthier snacks from the recipe section on hand.

Q: Can I swap meals around?

Yes. Flexibility is built into this plan to make it sustainable. Feel free to swap meals within the same week, as long as you maintain balance and stay within your recommended portion sizes.

Q: What about eating out?

Look for grilled, steamed, or baked foods without heavy sauces or breading. Always ask for no added salt. Choose sides like steamed vegetables instead of high-potassium options like baked potatoes or French fries.

Q: Can I drink coffee or tea?

Yes, in moderation. Stick to 1–2 cups per day and limit heavy creamers and added sugars. Remember, they are not a substitute for water—make sure you're drinking plenty of plain water too.

Q: Do I need to limit potassium or phosphorus?

You may need to be mindful, but Stage 3 usually doesn't require strict limits unless your blood tests show high levels. This plan naturally prioritizes lower-potassium foods and avoids high-phosphorus additives found in many processed foods.

Q: Why is controlling salt/sodium so important?

Controlling sodium helps manage blood pressure and fluid retention, which directly affects the workload of your kidneys. This plan focuses on fresh foods to give you control over your sodium intake.

60 DAY MEAL PLAN - MONTH 1

Day	Breakfast	Lunch	Dinner
1	Savannah Olive Scramble, p. 42	Shiraz Peach-Glazed Chicken Cutlets, p. 50	Mustard-Maple Rainbow Trout, p. 62
2	Burlington Cinnamon Oats, p. 45	Catalina Citrus Chicken & Peppers, p. 52	Guten Garden Egg-White Frittata, p. 64
3	Bismarck Vanilla Rice Bowl, p. 41	Mustard-Maple Rainbow Trout, p. 62	Soft Broccoli Cheddar Whisper, p. 75
4	Edison Egg White Hash, p. 35	Tuscany Tomato-Basil Chicken Piccata, p. 54	Gentle Beef Stew Sipper, p. 76
5	Abyss Blueberry Bliss, p. 48	Santa Fe Egg-White & Tofu Pepper Toss, p. 63	Catalina Cottage-Stuffed Mini Peppers, p. 65
6	Erie Sunny Tofu Hash, p. 40	Monterey Bay Tomato-Basil Flounder, p. 60	Big Bear Herb Seitan Sauté, p. 66
7	Charleston Cottage Cakes, p. 43	Sir James Rosemary Turkey Medallions, p. 50	Kyoto Ginger Egg-White Mushroom Stir-Fry, p. 64
8	Omaha Cottage Cheese Toast, p. 36	Nord Beef & Zucchini Sauté with Fried Egg, p. 55	Napa Chickpea-Zucchini Cakes, p. 67
9	Canton Banana Breakfast Melt, p. 37	Parisian Herb Beef & Bell Pepper Foil Packets, p. 57	Kyoto Ginger Egg-White Mushroom Stir-Fry, p. 64
10	Portland Sunrise Polenta, p. 38	Atlantic Breeze Lemon Cod, p. 58	Oklahoma Comfort Ginger-Beef, p. 56
11	Sunset Peach-Pine Splash, p. 48	Kyoto Ginger Egg-White Mushroom Stir-Fry, p. 64	Boulder BBQ Seitan & Pepper Skillet, p. 65
12	Lexington Light Bagel Stack, p. 46	Blue Ridge Apple-Sage Chicken, p. 54	Valletta White-Bean & Seitan Stew, p. 66
13	Route 66 Sunrise Smoothie, p. 47	Sesame-Lime Pollock Stir-Fry, p. 62	Guten Garden Egg-White Frittata, p. 64
14	Coral Bay Crunch Cup, p. 46	Santa Fe Chili-Lime Turkey Strips, p. 53	Cajun Red Drum Sauté, p. 61
15	Carmel Apple Rice Porridge, p. 35	Viennese Velvet Beef Strips, p. 55	Catalina Cottage-Stuffed Mini Peppers, p. 65
16	Reno Creamy Rice Frittata, p. 37	Oklahoma Comfort Ginger-Beef, p. 56	Citrus-Ginger Swai Fillet, p. 61

Day	Breakfast	Lunch	Dinner
17	Lato Cranberry Cooler, p. 49	Guten Garden Egg-White Frittata, p. 64	Big Bear Herb Seitan Sauté, p. 66
18	Wichita Whipped Egg Cups, p. 36	Tokyo Beef Lettuce Cups, p. 56	New England Light Clam Chowder, p. 75
19	Dayton Apple Oat Cup, p. 38	Cape Ann Herb-Crusted Cod, p. 58	Sir James Rosemary Turkey Medallions, p. 50
20	Mobile Mild Egg Salad Pita, p. 39	Gulf Coast Garlic Snapper Packets, p. 59	Santa Fe Egg-White & Tofu Pepper Toss, p. 63
21	Fresno Sunrise Rice Bowl, p. 40	Chesapeake Garden Tuna Patties, p. 60	Verona Egg-White Ricotta Zucchini Skillet, p. 63
22	Albany Almond Pancakes, p. 44	Maple Grove Dijon Chicken Tenders, p. 51	Valletta White-Bean & Seitan Stew, p. 66
23	Zagros Berry Cream Bowl, p. 44	Nashville Honey-Herb Turkey Patties, p. 52	Rustic Creamy Potato Bowl, p. 76
24	Backyard Strawberry Shortshake, p. 47	Verona Egg-White Ricotta Zucchini Skillet, p. 63	Boulder BBQ Seitan & Pepper Skillet, p. 65
25	Trenton Honey Cinnamon Quinoa, p. 42	Cajun Red Drum Sauté, p. 61	Guten Garden Egg-White Frittata, p. 64
26	Golden Fields Apple Pie Smoothie, p. 49	Catalina Cottage-Stuffed Mini Peppers, p. 65	Bangkok Basil Tofu-Seitan Stir-Fry, p. 67
27	Canton Banana Breakfast Melt, p. 37	Sir James Rosemary Turkey Medallions, p. 50	Boulder BBQ Seitan & Pepper Skillet, p. 65
28	Charleston Cottage Cakes, p. 43	Cape Ann Herb-Crusted Cod, p. 58	Bangkok Basil Tofu-Seitan Stir-Fry, p. 67
29	Reno Creamy Rice Frittata, p. 37	Bay-Island Coconut Catfish Skillet, p. 59	Kyoto Ginger Egg-White Mushroom Stir-Fry, p. 64
30	Charleston Cottage Cakes, p. 43	Shiraz Peach-Glazed Chicken Cutlets, p. 50	Verona Egg-White Ricotta Zucchini Skillet, p. 63

60 DAY MEAL PLAN - MONTH 2

Day	Breakfast	Lunch	Dinner
1	Reno Creamy Rice Frittata, **p. 37**	Nord Beef & Zucchini Sauté with Fried Egg, **p. 55**	Guten Garden Egg-White Frittata, **p. 64**
2	Charleston Cottage Cakes, **p. 43**	Tokyo Beef Lettuce Cups, **p. 56**	Kyoto Ginger Egg-White Mushroom Stir-Fry, **p. 64**
3	Erie Sunny Tofu Hash, **p. 40**	Sir James Rosemary Turkey Medallions, **p. 50**	Citrus-Ginger Swai Fillet, **p. 61**
4	Trenton Honey Cinnamon Quinoa, **p. 42**	Bay-Island Coconut Catfish Skillet, **p. 59**	Kyoto Ginger Egg-White Mushroom Stir-Fry, **p. 64**
5	Wichita Whipped Egg Cups, **p. 36**	Sesame-Lime Pollock Stir-Fry, **p. 55**	Guten Garden Egg-White Frittata, **p. 64**
6	Zagros Berry Cream Bowl, **p. 44**	Viennese Velvet Beef Strips, **p. 55**	Sir James Rosemary Turkey Medallions, **p. 50**
7	Mobile Mild Egg Salad Pita, **p. 39**	Maple Grove Dijon Chicken Tenders, **p. 51**	Catalina Cottage-Stuffed Mini Peppers, **p. 65**
8	Abyss Blueberry Bliss, **p. 48**	Verona Cranberry Chicken Sauté, **p. 53**	Big Bear Herb Seitan Sauté, **p. 66**
9	Maple Grove Egg Plate, **p. 43**	Atlantic Breeze Lemon Cod, **p. 58**	Santa Fe Egg-White & Tofu Pepper Toss, **p. 63**
10	Carmel Apple Rice Porridge, **p. 35**	Blue Ridge Apple-Sage Chicken, **p. 54**	Creamy Tomato Classic **p. 16**
11	Route 66 Sunrise Smoothie, **p. 47**	Mustard-Maple Rainbow Trout, **p. 62**	Boulder BBQ Seitan & Pepper Skillet, **p. 65**
12	Lexington Light Bagel Stack, **p. 46**	Oklahoma Comfort Ginger-Beef , **p. 56**	Rustic Creamy Potato Bowl, **p. 76**
13	Dayton Apple Oat Cup, **p. 38**	Nashville Honey-Herb Turkey Patties, **p. 52**	Valletta White-Bean & Seitan Stew, **p. 66**
14	Sonoma Soft Wrap Morning, **p. 45**	Cajun Red Drum Sauté, **p. 61**	Bangkok Basil Tofu-Seitan Stir-Fry, **p. 67**
15	Backyard Strawberry Shortshake, **p. 47**	Monterey Bay Tomato-Basil Flounder, **p. 60**	New England Light Clam Chowder, **p. 75**
16	Albany Almond Pancakes, **p. 44**	Catalina Citrus Chicken & Peppers, **p. 52**	Mustard-Maple Rainbow Trout, **p. 62**
17	Coral Bay Crunch Cup, **p. 46**	Citrus-Ginger Swai Fillet, **p. 61**	Sir James Rosemary Turkey Medallions, **p. 50**

Day	Breakfast	Lunch	Dinner
18	Portland Sunrise Polenta, p. 38	Key West Lime-Coconut Chicken Skillet, p. 51	Cajun Red Drum Sauté, p. 61
19	Edison Egg White Hash, p. 35	Parisian Herb Beef & Bell Pepper Foil Packets, p. 57	Chesapeake Garden Tuna Patties, p. 60
20	Lato Cranberry Cooler, p. 49	Santa Fe Chili-Lime Turkey Strips, p. 53	Boulder BBQ Seitan & Pepper Skillet, p. 65
21	Fresno Sunrise Rice Bowl, p. 40	Tuscany Tomato-Basil Chicken Piccata, p. 54	Guten Garden Egg-White Frittata, p. 64
22	Salem Peaches & Cream Bowl, p. 39	Gulf Coast Garlic Snapper Packets, p. 59	Gentle Beef Stew Sipper, p. 76
23	Lincoln Mild Cheese Toast, p. 41	Chesapeake Garden Tuna Patties, p. 60	Catalina Cottage-Stuffed Mini Peppers, p. 62
24	Omaha Cottage Cheese Toast, p. 36	Cape Ann Herb-Crusted Cod, p. 58	Sesame-Lime Pollock Stir-Fry, p. 62
25	Golden Fields Apple Pie Smoothie, p. 49	Tokyo Beef Lettuce Cups, p. 56	Soft Broccoli Cheddar Whisper, p. 75
26	Canton Banana Breakfast Melt, p. 37	Shiraz Peach-Glazed Chicken Cutlets, p. 50	Napa Chickpea-Zucchini Cakes, p. 67
27	Savannah Olive Scramble, p. 42	Mustard-Maple Rainbow Trout, p. 62	Oklahoma Comfort Ginger-Beef, p. 56
28	Sunset Peach-Pine Splash, p. 48	Oklahoma Comfort Ginger-Beef, p. 56	Valletta White-Bean & Seitan Stew, p. 66
29	Omaha Cottage Cheese Toast, p. 36	Cajun Red Drum Sauté, p. 61	Verona Egg-White Ricotta Zucchini Skillet , p. 63
30	Mobile Mild Egg Salad Pita, p. 39	Blue Ridge Apple-Sage Chicken, p. 54	Bangkok Basil Tofu-Seitan Stir-Fry, p. 67

5 Essential Steps for Seniors to Take Control of Stage 3 CKD

Step 1: The Stage 3 CKD Basics

Finding out you or a loved one has chronic kidney disease (CKD) c a n beoverwhelming, but understanding the basics can make things much less scary. CKD means your kidneys are slowly losing their ability to filter waste from your blood. There are five stages of CKD, based on how well your kidneys are still working. Your doctor can tell you which stage you're in after some simple blood tests.

In the early stages, most people feel totally normal with no symptoms at all. CKD can sneak up on you, so regular check-ups are important. As the diseaseworsens, symptoms like swelling, itchy skin, nausea, or changes in how often you urinate can start to show u p. That's why catching it early is such a big deal!

Here's the good news: you CAN manage CKD. There's no one-and-done cure, but changing how you eat and live can slow things down a lot—and help you feel better overall. Eating right for your kidneys can even help with other health issues linked to CKD, like high blood pressure or diabetes.

I want you to know that it's absolutely possible to lead a full, happy life with CKD. Making these changes now can help keep your symptoms at bay for years to come.

How This Book Will Help You

That's where this book comes in––it's here to make those changes feel doable.

This book is different from others on the same topic. It's made especially for you — seniors who deserve recipes as thoughtful, vibrant, and adaptable as you are.

We get straight to the heart of what matters: practical, real-life solutions tailored for your unique needs.

You get tools and ideas you can actually use every day. No overwhelming charts, no complicated medical lectures—just straightforward guidance that works.

Let me share a personal story. My husband faced a Stage 3 CKD diagnosis later in life. Like many seniors, he worried about his life, as he knew it was slipping away. But by making small, manageable changes—like the ones in this book—he reclaimed his health and joy.

This book's recipes are designed for

seniors: every meal takes **less than 30 minutes** to prepare, uses **five ingredients or fewer**, and requires **minimal kitchen equipment**. That means you can cook delicious, kidney-friendly meals without stress, fatigue, or the need for fancy gadgets. Some non perishable pantry items such as olive oil, water, dried herbs and honey are not counted in the 5 ingredients.

As you move through this cookbook, you'll find that managing CKD doesn't have to be complicated or overwhelming. These simple, tasty recipes and helpful tips are made for your pace, your kitchen, and your lifestyle.

Why? Because what works for a 30-year-old with CKD isn't always what you need in your 60s, 70s, or beyond. Your metabolism, energy, medications, and digestive system have changed. That's why this seniors' edition is here to make kidney-friendly eating easy, accessible, and enjoyable every day.

How to Use This Cookbook

◊ **Get the Basics Down**
Start by learning what Stage 3 CKD means and how food helps your kidneys.

◊ **Pick Your Favorites**
Explore easy recipes—from comforting soups to quick snacks—all with handy shopping lists.

◊ **Grab the Extras**
Use the printables and to stay organized and on track. $FIX

◊ **Team Up for Success**
Work with your health team and join our CKD facebook group for peer group support.

◊ **Take Small Steps**
Track your progress, start simple, and thrive big.

Let's keep it simple, stay motivated, and get going. Your new chapter starts now and I'm honored to join you.

What Is Stage 3 CKD?

Your kidneys are hardworking little organs—two bean-shaped filters working nonstop to clean about 120 to 150 quarts (about 114 to 142 liters) of blood every day. They keep your fluids balanced, help manage blood pressure, and remove waste through your urine.

When you have chronic kidney disease (CKD), your kidneys slowly lose some of their filtering power. Kidney disease is divided into five stages based on how well they're working. Stage 3 is the middle point—moderate loss of kidney function, with a GFR (glomerular filtration rate) between 30 and 59. Stage 3 is further divided into 3a (GFR 45–59%) and 3b (GFR 30–44%), with 3b indicating more severe impairment. GFR is a number your doctor calculates using a blood test,

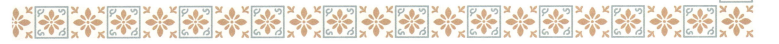

age, gender, and race—it tells you how well your kidneys filter waste.

At stage 3, your kidneys are not working as well as they should, but the good news is this stage gives you a critical window for early action. Catching it here means you can slow the damage and keep your kidneys functioning longer. Your kidneys are like coffee filters: if the filter gets clogged, the coffee doesn't drip as well. But if you catch it early, you can avoid a full clog and keep enjoying your cu p.

In Stage 3, waste and fluids build up more than usual, which can lead to symptoms. However,adjusting your lifestyle and diet will give your kidneys a break. Acting early is your best bet to keep feeling good and will help protect your independence.

Common Symptoms and What to Watch For

In early stages of CKD, many people feel completely normal. That's why it's called a "silent" disease—it sneaks up quietly. But as kidney function dips into Stage 3, you might start noticing some signs:

◊ **Fatigue: Feeling more tired than usual, even with enough rest.**

The science behind this: This happens because damaged kidneys produce less erythropoietin, a hormone that signals the bone marrow to make red blood cells. Fewer red blood cells mean less oxygen delivery to tissues, causing fatigue.

◊ **Swelling: Puffy ankles, feet, or**

hands caused by fluid buildu p.

◊ **Changes in urination: More or less frequent trips to the bathroom, foamy or dark urine.**

◊ **Itchy skin or rashes: Waste buildup can irritate your skin.**

◊ **Nausea or loss of appetite: Feeling queasy or not hungry.**

◊ **Shortness of breath: This symptom occurs if fluid builds up in your lungs.**

◊ **Trouble concentrating or dizziness: This occurs from imbalanced minerals or anemia.**

Noticing any of these? It's important to bring them up with your doctor at your next visit. Simple blood and urine tests to check your GFR and protein levels in urine will help guide your treatment.

Remember, symptoms can be subtle or occur due to other health issues. That's why regular check-ups and honest talks with your healthcare team are so important. Don't wait for symptoms to get worse—early awareness is your best defense.

CKD Progression: What You Can Influence

Here's some hopeful news: while there's no cure for CKD, you can take meaningful steps to slow it down. What you eat and how you live matter more than you might think. Choosing kidney-friendly foods and making healthy lifestyle changes protect your kidneys while they also improve how you feel day to day.

Eating well for your kidneys can also help manage health issues like high blood pressure or diabetes. These conditions often go hand-in-hand with CKD and can speed up kidney damage if left unchecked. That's why a balanced approach to diet and lifestyle is key.

Besides food, other parts of your daily routine can influence your kidney health. Staying active (even gentle movement counts), getting good sleep, managing your weight, reducing stress, and avoiding cigarettes and excessive alcohol all support your kidneys and overall well-being. These small choices contribute healthover time, helping you feel stronger and more energetic.

Doctors and dietitians use some medical terms—like "glomerular filtration rate" (GFR) or urine protein levels—to track how your kidneys are doing. I won't get too technical here, but know these tests help your healthcare team adjust your plan so it fits you perfectly. Staying in touch with them and reporting how you feel is one of your best tools.

Myths vs. Facts

◊ **We will debunk the "You can't eat anything" myth and other common fears**

◊ **Clarify misconceptions around protein, fruit, and phosphorus**

One of the biggest worries when you hear "kidney disease" is protein. For decades, many believed eating less protein was best to protect your kidneys. That advice stuck around so long it's hard to shake—but modern science tells a more balanced story.

Cutting protein too low can actually hurt, especially for older adults. Protein keeps muscles strong. Too little protein means weaker muscles, more risk of injury and falls, and slower recovery.

Who truly needs to limit protein? Usually only people with very high protein in their urine or quickly worsening kidney function—your doctor will let you know if that's you.

For most people with Stage 3 CKD, the key is to get the right amount of protein, not too little or too much. About 0.27 – 0.36 grams per pound of body weight or 0.6-0.8 grams of protein per Kg of body weight daily is a good target. For example, a person weighing 150 pounds (68 kg) would aim for 0.3g/lb which is about 45 grams of protein per day.

It's also helpful to focus on where your protein comes from. Plant-based sources like beans, nuts, and tofu are easier on the kidneys, but lean animal proteins like skinless chicken, fish, or eggs can be included too. Balance and variety make your meals both nourishing and enjoyable.

Besides protein, many people worry about **fruits and potassium**. It's true

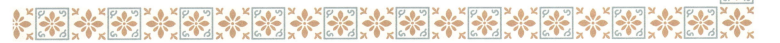

some fruits are higher in potassium (like bananas), which can be a concern for kidney health, but plenty of delicious options—like apples, berries, and grapes—fit well in a kidney-friendly diet. **Phosphorus** is another mineral that can sneak into processed foods and sodas, so choosing fresh, whole foods is usually safer. The key is knowing what to watch for—not cutting everything out. You can still enjoy great meals and snacks that support your kidneys.

Remember, your healthcare team or dietitian will help fine-tune your diet based on your unique health. Don't hesitate to ask questions—they're your partners in this journey.

Step 1 Recap:

◊ **Stage 3 CKD Overview:** It's a moderate loss of kidney function (GFR 30–59), often with no early symptoms—early detection through routine tests and making lifestyle changes are keys to slowing progression.

◊ **Manageable With Lifestyle Changes:** CKD isn't curable but can be managed effectively through diet, exercise, sleep, and avoiding harmful habits like smoking or excess alcohol.

◊ **Symptoms to Watch:** As CKD progresses, watch for fatigue, swelling, itchy skin, urination changes, nausea, and shortness of breath—regular check-ups are essential.

◊ **Practical, Senior-Friendly Cookbook:** This guide offers quick, simple recipes (≤30 mins, ≤5 ingredients) tailored for seniors, making kidney-friendly eating easy and stress-free.

◊ **Myths Debunked:** You don't have to cut out all protein—balanced intake is important; plant and lean proteins are kidney-friendly, and many fruits are still safe with proper guidance.

Step 2: Know Your Nutritional Numbers

Understanding the key nutrients that affect kidney health makes managing CKD easier and less intimidating. Let's break down the essentials — protein, sodium, potassium, phosphorus, fluids, and calories — so you can make smart, practical choices every day.

Protein – Not Too Much, Not Too Little

Protein helps keep muscles strong and supports overall health, but too much or too little can be tough on your kidneys.

We introduced this a little earlier, but it's worth repeating. **Aim for about 0.5 grams of protein per pound (or 1 grams per kilogram) of body weight daily.** For example, someone weighing 68 kg (150 lbs) should target roughly 68 grams of protein per day.

Plant and animal proteins both count:

◊ **Lean meats like skinless chicken,**

fish, and turkey are great choices.

◊ **Plant options like tofu, beans, nuts, and lentils are foods thekidneys love, plus they add healthy fiber.**

◊ **Portion guide: 1 oz (28g) cooked meat or poultry = 7g protein; ½ cup cooked beans ~2g protein; 125g (½ cup) cooked tofu = 10g protein.**

If your urine shows high protein or kidney function worsens quickly, your doctor may adjust your intake.

Pro Tip: Using a kitchen scale to weigh portions helps take the guesswork out of protein control.

2.2 Sodium – The Sneaky Saboteur

Sodium (salt) is often hiding where you least expect it — canned soups, processed foods, frozen meals, and salty snacks. Too much sodium can raise blood pressure and make your kidneys work harder. This in turn can lead to high blood pressure that needs medication. And all medications stress the kidneys in their own ways.

Keep your sodium intake under 2,000 mg per day. To put that in perspective, 1 teaspoon of salt contains about 2,300 mg sodium — so every pinch counts!

Label savvy:

◊ **"Low sodium" means less than 140 mg per serving.**

◊ **Avoid items with over 500 mg per serving. That one serving could use up one-fourth of the daily quota for sodium!**

◊ **Check ingredient lists for hidden sodium additives.**

Instead of salt, use fresh herbs, lemon juice, garlic, and spices to add flavor without extra sodium.

2.3 Potassium & Phosphorus – Hidden Challenges

Both potassium and phosphorus can sneak into your diet unnoticed but cause real trouble for kidney health if not monitored.

Potassium helps muscles and nerves work, but too much can affect your heart rhythm. Aim for about **2,000 mg per day,** but your doctor may set a different target. Avoid high-potassium foods like bananas, potatoes, tomatoes, and oranges; instead, enjoy apples, berries, grapes, and lettuce.

Also, read the label to see if a food contains any potassium additives like (potassium acetate, or potassium alginate etc...). If it does, choose something else.

Phosphorus supports bones but builds up when kidneys struggle. Keep phosphorus around **1,000 mg daily.** Watch out for processed foods and sodas, which often contain **phosphorus additives labeled with "phos" in the ingredients** (e.g., phosphoric acid or sodium tripolyphosphate).

Quick tip: Fresh, whole foods are generally lower in hidden phosphorus and potassium.

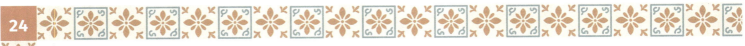

2.4 Fluids & Hydration

Your kidneys balance fluids carefully. In most cases with early to moderate CKD, fluid limits are unnecessary. But if swelling, high blood pressure, or low urine output occur, your healthcare provider may recommend a fluid limit.

Drink steadily throughout the day, choosing mostly water. If plain water feels boring, add cucumber slices or a sprig of mint for a refreshing twist.

Avoid sodas, sugary drinks, and some teas with high potassium or caffeine.

Watch for signs of dehydration: dry mouth, dark urine, dizziness, or headaches.

2.5 Calories: The Fuel Your Body Needs

Calories give your body energy and help maintain muscle. Most adults with CKD need about **30–35 calories per kilogram of body weight daily.** For example, a 68 kg (150 lb) person requires roughly **2,000 to 2,400 calories each day.**

If weight changes suddenly, track your intake and set up an appointment with your healthcare professional. The goal is to provide enough energy without stressing your kidneys.

You can use online tools like the National Institute of Diabetes and Digestive and Kidney Diseases (NIDDK) Body Weight Planner for personalized calorie needs.

https://www.niddk.nih.gov/bwp

Step 2 Recap:

◊ **Protein Balance Is Key:** Aim for ~0.3g per pound of body weight daily; both plant and lean animal proteins are okay. Too little protein weakens muscles while too much stresses kidneys.

◊ **Limit Sodium Intake:** Keep sodium under 2,000 mg/day. Avoid processed foods and use herbs/spices instead of salt. Read labels for sodium content and discover the hidden additives.

◊ **Watch Potassium & Phosphorus:** Limit high-potassium foods (bananas, tomatoes) and high-phosphorus items (processed foods, sodas). Opt for fresh, whole foods and check for additives.

◊ **Stay Hydrated Smartly:** Most Stage 3 CKD patients don't need strict fluid limits unless swelling or high BP occurs. Choose mostly water and avoid sugary or high-potassium drinks.

◊ **Meet Calorie Needs:** Aim for 30–35 calories/kg of body weight daily to maintain energy and muscle. Adjust intake with guidance if weight changes significantly.

Step 3: To eat or not to eat

Goal: Empower food choices through lists, visuals, and practical swaps.

3.1 Kidney-Friendly Foods to Enjoy

When it comes to kidney health,

knowing what to add to your plate is just as important as what to avoid. The following foods are low in sodium and phosphorus, with moderate potassium—gentler on the kidneys, budget-conscious, and senior-friendly:
 Top Picks for Everyday Meals:

- ◊ **Grains & Carbs: White rice, pasta, plain white or wheat bread, unsalted crackers, and flour tortillas.**

- ◊ **Protein (Fresh is Best): Skinless chicken, turkey, fish, eggs, tofu, and unsalted nuts (small amounts).**

- ◊ **Dairy & Substitutes: Plain milk, unflavored soy milk, unsweetened Greek yogurt, low-sodium cheese.**

- ◊ **Veggies: Carrots, green beans, cucumbers, lettuce, bell peppers, cabbage, cauliflower (fresh or frozen).**

- ◊ **Fruits: Apples, berries, grapes, peaches or pears (fresh or canned in water or juice).**

- ◊ **Healthy Fats: Olive oil, grass-fed butter and ghee, avocado, walnuts, flaxseed oil.**

- ◊ **Seasonings: Lemon juice, vinegar, garlic, fresh herbs, salt-free spice mixes.**

These are practical, affordable staples you can find in most grocery stores—and they're easy to prep whether you're cooking for yourself or someone you love.

- ◊ **Best bets" list (low sodium, low phosphorus, moderate potassium)**

- ◊ **Budget- and senior-friendly items**

3.2 Foods to Limit (Or Watch Closely)

Some foods hit the kidneys like a speed bum p. They're either high in sodium, contain phosphate or potassium additives, or are just too processed.
⚠️ Use With Caution:

- ◊ **Canned & Processed Foods: Canned soups, beans, vegetables (unless low/no salt), boxed mixes, frozen meals.**

- ◊ **Processed Meats: Bacon, hot dogs, sausages, lunch meats, ham, pepperoni.**

- ◊ **Dairy & Cheeses: American cheese, processed slices, cottage cheese, cheese spreads.**

- ◊ **Snacks: Salted chips, microwave popcorn, flavored crackers, trail mixes with salted nuts.**

- ◊ **Condiments & Extras: Soy sauce, BBQ sauce, ketchup, salad dressings, bouillon cubes.**

- ◊ **Phosphorus Additives: Look for ingredients with the letters "phos" in the word—like phosphoric acid, sodium phosphate, etc.**

- ◊ **Potassium Additives: Skip anything with potassium chloride, potassium citrate, or potassium phosphate.**

👍 Smart Substitutes:

- ◊ **Use fresh or frozen vegetables over canned.**

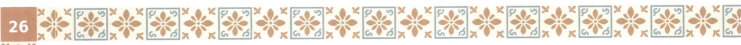

- ◊ Try **grilled meats** instead of cured or smoked ones.
- ◊ Replace **cheese** with avocado or homemade hummus.
- ◊ Use **herbs, lemon, and garlic** in place of salt-based seasonings.

3.3 Smart Ingredient Swaps

Living with CKD doesn't mean bland meals. Make clever swaps that protect your kidneys and still bring flavor to the table.

Salt Swap Ideas:

- ◊ Use **garlic, onion powder, fresh herbs, lemon zest, or salt-free blends** instead of table salt.

- ◊ Avoid **seasoned salts, bouillon, or spice mixes** with sodium.

Choose Cleaner Proteins

Conventional meats often contain hormones, additives, and residues that your kidneys—and your whole body—don't need. These additives and residues put extra work on your kidneys by having to be removed from your body. A small shift in choosing proteins without them can make a big difference.

- ◊ **Look for grass-fed, pasture-raised meats**
- ◊ **Choose wild-caught fish—** never farmed or genetically modified
- ◊ **Go for ghee or butter from grass-fed cows,** which have better fat profiles

Avoid home-raised or farmed fish that are often fed preservatives and synthetic hormones.

Dairy Swaps:

- ◊ Choose **unsweetened soy milk** or **rice milk** over cow's milk.
- ◊ Use **plain Greek yogurt** instead of sour cream or cream cheese.

Smart Bread Picks & Fermented Friends

- ◊ **Sourdough bread** is easier on digestion and often lower in additives and potassium than commercial whole grain breads.
- ◊ **Fermented foods** like sauerkraut (rinse before using), kimchi (low-sodium versions), or kefir (in moderation) can boost your gut health—and a healthy gut supports better kidney and immune function.
- ◊ Opt for **low-sodium tortillas or unsalted crackers** as side options. Choose minimally processed versions without added sodium or phosphorus.
- ◊ Go for **plain white bread or pasta** (low in potassium/phosphorus) over whole wheat or multigrain unless guided otherwise by your doctor.

A thriving gut microbiome can ease inflammation, boost nutrient absorption, and help your body work more efficiently—including kidney filtration.

🧴 Fats & Spreads:

Not all oils are created equal. Most commercial cooking oils are refined and can clog up your system—literally. The kidneys are filtration organs, and healthy fats make their job easier, not harder.

- ◊ **Cold-pressed avocado oil** (neutral flavor, great for high-heat cooking)
- ◊ **Cold-pressed olive oil** (ideal for dressings or sautéing)
- ◊ **Unrefined, cold-pressed coconut oil** (best in moderation, especially for baking)
- ◊ **Grass-fed tallow or ghee** (stable at high heat and free of additives)
- ◊ **Try nut butters** (unsalted, 1 tbsp or 15g at a time) for flavor without the extra sodium.

🔧 Bonus Tip: Mayonnaise Matters

Many store-bought mayos hide preservatives, sugar, and additives that aren't kidney- or heart-friendly.

- ◊ ✅ Choose **avocado oil mayo** (check the ingredients—no soybean oil or preservatives).

- ◊ ✅ Or make your own mayo with **egg yolks, lemon juice, and cold-pressed oil**—simple, wholesome, and tasty!

3.4 Pantry, non-refrigerated, shelf-stable ingredients

These pantry staples are your kitchen's secret weapons—versatile, shelf-stable ingredients that add flavor, texture, and balance to almost any dish. From oils and vinegars to spices, dried herbs, and baking basics, they're essentials you'll use again and again. Since they're common, long-lasting, and used in small amounts, they don't count toward the 5 ingredients in each recipe—just think of them as your always-ready support crew that makes simple cooking even better.

🧂 Seasonings, Herbs & Spices

- ◊ **Sea salt** (fine or coarse)
- ◊ **Black pepper** (freshly ground or pre-ground)
- ◊ **White pepper**
- ◊ **Garlic powder** (not garlic salt)
- ◊ **Onion powder**
- ◊ **Dried herbs:**
- ◊ **Basil**
- ◊ **Oregano**
- ◊ **Thyme**
- ◊ **Parsley**
- ◊ **Dill**
- ◊ **Rosemary**
- ◊ **Spices:**
- ◊ **Cinnamon**
- ◊ **Paprika**
- ◊ **Cumin**
- ◊ **Nutmeg**
- ◊ **Salt substitute** (only if potassium and phosphorus-free)
- ◊ **Vanilla extract** (alcohol-based or alcohol-free)

🧴 Oils & Fats

◊ Olive oil (cooking)

◊ Extra virgin olive oil (for dressing/finishing)

◊ Grass-fed butter (shelf-stable short-term or if clarified)

🥛 Liquids & Vinegars

◊ Water (for cooking, naturally shelf-stable)

◊ Vinegars:

◊ White vinegar

◊ Apple cider vinegar

◊ Red wine vinegar

◊ Lemon or lime juice (bottled, shelf-stable until opened)

🍯 Sweeteners

◊ Honey

◊ White sugar

◊ Maple syrup (pure, small amounts)

🥫 Pantry & Dry Goods

◊ Canned plum tomatoes

🍞 Baking Essentials

◊ Baking powder (low sodium and aluminum-free preferred)

◊ Baking soda (low sodium)

Dressings

◊ Homemade mayo (recipe in the book)

Step 3 Recap:

◊ **Kidney-Friendly Foods to Enjoy:** Focus on fresh or frozen low-sodium items like white rice, lean meats, tofu, carrots, apples, olive oil, and herbs—easy to prep and gentle on kidneys.

◊ **Foods to Limit or Avoid:** Cut back on processed, high-sodium, and additive-heavy items (e.g., canned soups, processed meats, American cheese, sauces, and snacks with "phos" or potassium additives).

◊ **Smart Ingredient Swaps:** Use herbs for flavors instead of salt. Choose wild-caught fish and grass-fed meats. Use soy milk over cow's milk, sourdough over whole wheat, and kidney-friendly oils like olive or avocado.

◊ **Shelf-Stable Pantry Staples:** Stock up on safe seasonings, oils, vinegars, and vbaking basics—these don't count toward recipe limits and add flexibility and flavor to meals.

◊ **Flavor Without Compromise:** Enjoy spreads like avocado oil mayo or nut butters, and use fermented foods (low-sodium) like sauerkraut or kefir in moderation to support gut and kidney health.

STEP 4: Food habits for Kidney Health

4.1 Know Your Portions: A Plate That Protects Your Kidneys

Big portions can sneak up on the plates

of even the best of us, especially during family meals or holidays. The good news? Portion control is really based on smart balance 'rules', not hunger.

Try the Balanced Plate Method:

◊ ½ plate = low-potassium vegetables (e.g., green beans, carrots, bell peppers)

◊ ¼ plate = lean protein (like 75g of grilled chicken or 125g of tofu)

◊ ¼ plate = kidney-friendly carbs (such as white rice or pasta)

Quick Trick: A serving of meat or fish should be about the size of a deck of cards (85g), and ½ cup of cooked rice or pasta is roughly a handful (about 100g).

Moderation is what keeps the kidneys from working overtime. Once you're familiar with the plate method, it becomes second nature—like riding a bike, but tastier.

⏰ 4.2 Timing Meals & Smart Snacking

Spacing meals throughout the day helps stabilize blood sugar and energy—especially important if there's diabetes involved. It also helps avoid the "I'm starving—what's closest?" trap that often leads to poor choices.

Tips for Gentle Meal Timing:

◊ **Eat every 3–4 hours to prevent energy dips and nausea.**

◊ **Don't skip meals—especially breakfast.**

◊ **Have small, steady snacks if there's a long gap between meals.**

👩‍🍳 4.3 Kitchen Tips for Seniors: Cook Once, Eat Twice

Keep Prep Simple

◊ **Use pre-chopped veggies or frozen options.**

◊ **Try slow cookers or one-pot meals to reduce clean-u p.**

◊ **Cut down time and effort by planning ahead with batch cooking.**

Tools That Make Life Easier:

● **Jar openers** and **grip pads** for arthritis

● **Electric can openers** and **chopping aids**

● **Ergonomic knives** and **stools** for seated prep

If energy's low, cook in short bursts and freeze portions. Make the freezer your friend—it doesn't mind leftovers.

4.4 Cracking Nutrition Labels (The Easy Way)

Nutrition labels might look like puzzles, but they hold kidney-saving clues. Here's how to shop smarter:
What to Look For:

◊ **Sodium: Aim for under 140 mg per serving. Anything above 500 mg? Best left on the shelf.**

◊ **Phosphorus:** Not always listed. Check for ingredients with **"phos"** (e.g., phosphate, phosphoric acid).

◊ **Potassium:** If listed, stay aware of your daily target (usually around 2,000 mg/day). Watch out for ingredients like **potassium chloride** or **potassium phosphate**.

Quick Example:

Two cans of beans—one has **300 mg sodium**, the other has just **15 mg** and no phosphate additives. The lower-sodium, additive-free version is your kidney's best friend.

🛒 **Label Detective Rule:** When in doubt, the fresher the food, the fewer the surprises.

Nutrient Claims: What to Look For

Some food labels highlight helpful claims like:

"Very low sodium"

"Low sodium"

"Reduced salt"

These aren't just buzzwords; manufacturers must follow strict guidelines to use them. Let these labels be your shortcut to making smarter, kidney-friendly choices.

Dining Out with Confidence

Having CKD doesn't mean missing out on restaurants or celebrations—it just means being a little more mindful with your choices. With a few simple swaps and questions, you can enjoy meals out while keeping your kidneys supported.

◊ 📞 **Call Ahead When You Can** - a quick phone call can ease a lot of worry. Call during slower hours and ask: Can dishes be prepared without added salt or sauces on the side?

◊ **Ask the server** if dishes can be made without added salt, sauces, or seasoning blends. And call beforehand to ask.

◊ **Choose wisely:** go for grilled, baked, poached, or steamed options instead of fried or smothered.

◊ **Control portions** by sharing a dish or boxing up half to enjoy the next day.

◊ **Skip the salt traps**—fries, pickles, or heavily seasoned sides—and ask if you can substitute with plain vegetables or rice.

A little planning makes the whole experience more relaxed—and much more enjoyable.

Social Events: Celebrate, Don't Stress

Just because you're watching your diet doesn't mean the party's over. At get-togethers:

◊ Offer to bring a **kidney-friendly dish** so there's something safe (and tasty!) on the table.

◊ Don't show up starving—have a light snack (like deviled eggs) beforehand so you can make clearer food choices.

◊ Focus on the people, not just the

food. Linger over conversations, share stories, laugh—these are the real heart of any gathering.

◊ One less-than-perfect meal won't undo your progress. It's your long-term habits that matter most.

Remember: joy is part of the treatment plan. Your health matters, but so does living a full, connected life.

Step 4 Recap:

◊ **Balanced Plate Method:** Use ½ plate for low-potassium veggies, ¼ for lean protein, and ¼ for kidney-friendly carbs; watch portion sizes to avoid overloading kidneys.

◊ **Meal Timing & Snacking:** Eat every 3–4 hours, don't skip meals (especially breakfast), and include light snacks to maintain energy and avoid poor food choices.

◊ **Simple Cooking for Seniors:** Use tools and shortcuts (like frozen veggies, one-pot meals, batch cooking) to make cooking easier and more efficient.

◊ **Reading Nutrition Labels:** Choose low-sodium (under 140 mg), avoid phosphate additives, and watch potassium content; fresh food is usually safer.

◊ **Dining Out & Socializing Smart:** Call ahead, request low-salt options, manage portions, and

focus on enjoying company—not just the food. Joyful living supports kidney health too.

Step 5: A fun and supportive CKD lifestyle

Work With Your Doctor, Not Just For Them

Managing Stage 3 CKD is not a solo mission. Your care team is your health GPS. Regular check-ups are more than routine—they're vital. Your doctor will be regularly monitoring key labs like:

◊ eGFR (to track kidney function),

◊ Creatinine, Potassium, Phosphorus

◊ Protein in the urine

◊ Bring thoughtful questions to every appointment. A few good ones:

◊ "Am I getting the right amount of protein?"

◊ "Is my potassium in the safe range?"

◊ "Should we tweak anything based on my latest labs?"

Most importantly, ask for a referral to a **renal dietitian**—someone who can craft a food plan that fits your stage, your symptoms, and your taste buds. This specialist can help adjust your meals without draining the joy from your plate.

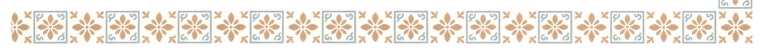

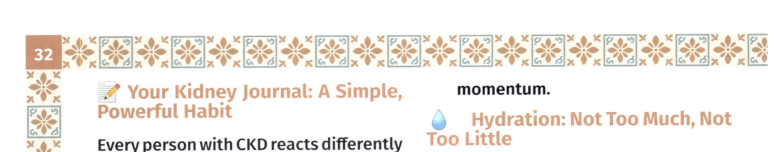

📝 Your Kidney Journal: A Simple, Powerful Habit

Every person with CKD reacts differently to foods, fluids, and routines. One of the smartest things you can do? Keep track.

Record daily:

◊ **What you ate (rough notes are fine but do include portion sizes)**

◊ **How much fluid you drank**

◊ **Any symptoms** like swelling, fatigue, or nausea

Practical tip: A basic notebook or calendar will do. Even writing down just 2–3 lines per day gives you—and your care team—valuable clues. It's like having a health diary that talks back.

Over time, this log helps uncover what's working, what's not, and when you might need to pivot. A small effort that brings big peace of mind.

🧠 Mindset First: Celebrate the Small Wins

Living with Stage 3 CKD is about progressive upgrades, not perfection. Shifting focus from what's off-limits to what supports your health makes the journey easier—and far more satisfying.

Each small win counts:

◊ **Choosing water instead of sugary drinks**

◊ **Cooking a meal at home**

◊ **Asking questions when dining out**

◊ **These aren't minor steps—they're**
momentum.

💧 Hydration: Not Too Much, Not Too Little

Unless your healthcare provider says

otherwise, aim for **6–8 cups (1.5–2 liters)** of fluid per day. Water is your best bet—simple, safe, and kidney-friendly.

Older adults may not feel thirst as strongly, so sipping steadily throughout the day helps keep things balanced. Try keeping a water glass bottle close and take small drinks regularly, rather than large gulps all at once. And do remember that you do not want to consume plasticized water, which is water stored in plastic bottles.

🧘 How to Feel Good Living With CKD

Chronic kidney disease affects your kidneys and how you feel every day. That's why feeling good with CKD goes beyond just food choices. The way you move, rest, and handle stress all play a powerful role in protecting your health and energy.

The good news? You don't need a gym membership, fancy gear, or meditation retreats. Just small daily choices that help your body and mood feel stronger and more supported.

🚶 Gentle Movement = Big Benefits

Even light physical activity helps your circulation, muscle strength, digestion, and blood pressure—all of which support kidney health. Don't think of this as "exercise." Think of it as gentle movement your body enjoys.

Try This:

- ◊ A 10–15 minute walk around your block or hallway
- ◊ Chair stretches or seated leg lifts during TV time
- ◊ Light gardening or dancing in your kitchen to a favorite song

Movement keeps your body flexible, your joints looser, and your spirits lifted. Always check with your doctor before starting something new.

🌿 Simple Stress Relief

Stress can raise your blood pressure, affect your sleep, and even impact your appetite and energy. Finding calm moments each day is one of the healthiest habits you can build.

Try This:

- ◊ Deep breathing: Inhale for 4 seconds, hold for 4, exhale for 4 (repeat 3–5 times).
- ◊ Listen to soft music, read, pray, or knit—anything that soothes your mind.
- ◊ Sit quietly with a cup of tea and look outside—it counts!

You don't need to "empty your mind"—just give it a break.

😴 Better Sleep, Happier Kidneys

Sleep is your body's reset button. It's when your kidneys and other systems repair, balance, and recover. But many seniors struggle with staying asleep or falling asleep easily.

Try This:

- ◊ Wind down 30 minutes before bed—turn off screens and dim the lights.
- ◊ Take a warm bath or shower to relax your muscles.
- ◊ Avoid heavy meals, caffeine, or large drinks late in the day.
- ◊ Keep your bedroom cool, dark, and quiet.

If you wake often or feel unrested, bring it up with your doctor—there may be solutions that don't involve medication.

Step 5 Recap:

- ◊ **Partner with Your Doctor:** Collaborate on care, monitor key labs (eGFR, creatinine, potassium, etc.), and ask for a renal dietitian referral.
- ◊ **Track Your Health:** Keep a simple daily journal of food, fluids, and symptoms to identify patterns and guide care adjustments.
- ◊ **Adopt a Positive Mindset:** Celebrate small wins like healthy food choices and asking informed questions—progress matters more than perfection.
- ◊ **Hydrate Wisely:** Aim for 6–8 cups of fluid daily unless told otherwise; sip steadily to stay balanced, especially if thirst is reduced.
- ◊ **Support Body and Mind:** Prioritize gentle movement, daily stress relief, and good sleep habits to boost energy, mood, and kidney

function.

Are you finding this book helpful so far?

I'D LOVE TO HEAR WHAT YOU THINK.

I personally read every review, and your feedback means the world to me.It only takes 30 seconds to leave a reivew.

It truly makes a huge difference for a small author like me, and it helps other CKD warriors discover this book too.

Here's how you can leave a review::

- **Option 1: Scan the QR code to go straight to the review page. (you will be asked to login to your Amazon Account)**
- Option 2: Go to your Amazon orders,

find this book, and click "Write a product review."

Option 3: Search for the book title on Amazon, scroll down to the "Customer Reviews" section, and click "Write a Review."

Once you're there, choose a star rating, a quick story about your experience, and submit! Anything you've learned so far! Only a sentence or two is also ok.

THAT'S IT!

Thank you so much and hope to see you in our grou p.

/ MARIANNE <3

Now it's time to turn the page and dig into the quick and delicious 5 ingredient recipes!

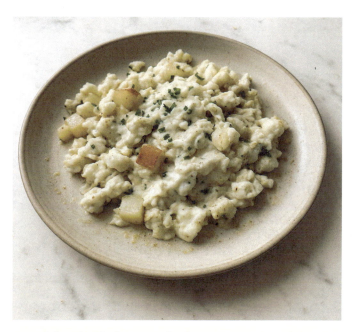

Edison Egg White Hash

Servings	Prep Time	Cook time	PROTEIN	PHOSPHORUS	SODIUM	POTASSIUM
1	7'	10'	MID	LOW	LOW	LOW

INGREDIENTS
- About 4 large egg whites (140 g)
- 3 Tbsp peeled cooked potato (45 g)
- 2 Tbsp cooked white rice (25 g)
- 2 Tbsp low-sodium cream cheese (25 g)
- 2 Tbsp olive oil (30 ml) (pantry)
- Fresh chives or parsley (optional)

DIRECTIONS
1. Combine egg whites, diced potato, and rice in a bowl.
2. Heat olive oil in a skillet over medium heat.
3. Pour mixture into skillet; scramble gently until almost set.
4. Stir in cream cheese until creamy and heated through.
5. Garnish with herbs and serve warm.

Nutritional Info (per serving)
Calories: ~505 kcal | Protein: ~20.6 g | Potassium: ~352 mg | Phosphorus: ~85 mg | Sodium: ~190 mg | Fat: ~33 g | Carbs: ~22 g | Cholesterol: 0 mg | Oxalates: ~1.4 mg

Creativity TWIST:
Add a pinch of smoked paprika or cumin to the scramble for a smoky, warming flavor.

Carmel Apple Rice Porridge

Servings	Prep Time	Cook time	PROTEIN	PHOSPHORUS	SODIUM	POTASSIUM
1	6'	10'	MID	LOW	LOW	LOW

INGREDIENTS
- ½ cup cooked white rice (60g)
- ⅔ cup rice milk, unsweetened (140g)
- ½ medium apple, peeled and diced (60g)
- ⅓ cup egg whites (80g)
- 1 Tbsp honey (21g) (Pantry)
- 1 Tbsp olive oil (15g) (Pantry)

DIRECTIONS
1. In a saucepan, combine cooked rice, rice milk, and diced apple. Bring to a gentle simmer over medium heat.
2. Stir in egg whites and cook gently, stirring constantly, until the mixture thickens and becomes creamy, about 2–3 minutes.
3. Remove from heat and swirl in honey and olive oil. Serve warm.

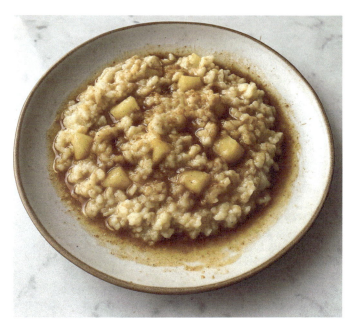

Nutritional Info (per serving)
Calories: ~520 kcal | Protein: ~20g | Potassium: ~260mg | Phosphorus: ~75mg | Sodium: ~110mg | Fat: ~15g | Carbs: ~55g | Cholesterol: 0mg | Oxalates: ~1.8mg

Creativity TWIST:
Try adding a pinch of cinnamon or nutmeg for a warm spice note.

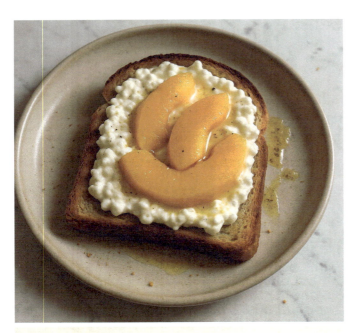

Omaha Cottage Cheese Toast

Servings	Prep Time	Cook time	PROTEIN	PHOSPHORUS	SODIUM	POTASSIUM
1	4'	4'	MID	LOW	LOW	LOW

INGREDIENTS
- 1 slice low-sodium white bread (32 g)
- 140 g low-sodium cottage cheese (2% fat)
- 60 g peeled canned peaches (in juice, drained)
- 2 Tbsp olive oil (30 mL) (including 1 Tbsp extra virgin olive oil) (Pantry)
- Fresh mint or cinnamon (optional)

DIRECTIONS
1. Toast the bread slice until golden and crisp.
2. Spread cottage cheese evenly over warm toast.
3. Layer sliced peaches on top of the cottage cheese.
4. Drizzle olive oil evenly over toast and toppings.
5. Sprinkle fresh mint leaves or dash of cinnamon if desired. Serve immediately.

Nutritional Info (per serving)
Calories: 480 kcal | Protein: 18.6 g | Potassium: 254 mg | Phosphorus: 158 mg | Sodium: 271 mg | Fat: 31.2 g |Carbs: 26 g | Cholesterol: 14 mg | Oxalates: 0.9 mg

Creativity TWIST:
Try swapping peaches for canned pears or pineapple for a different fruity flavor.

Wichita Whipped Egg Cups

Servings	Prep Time	Cook time	PROTEIN	PHOSPHORUS	SODIUM	POTASSIUM
1	5'	8'	MID	LOW	LOW	LOW

INGREDIENTS
- About About 4 large egg whites (120 g)
- 3 1/2 Tbsp cooked white rice (50 g)
- 2 Tbsp peeled cooked carrot, mashed (30 g)
- 2 Tbsp olive oil (30 mL) (Pantry)
- Chives or black pepper (optional)

DIRECTIONS
1. Preheat oven to 350°F (175°C). Lightly grease 2 muffin cups with olive oil.
2. In a bowl, mix egg whites, cooked rice, mashed carrot, and 1 Tbsp olive oil until combined.
3. Divide mixture evenly between muffin cups. Bake for 8 minutes or until set and firm.
4. Drizzle remaining 1 Tbsp olive oil over the baked cups. Garnish with chives or black pepper if desired. Serve warm.

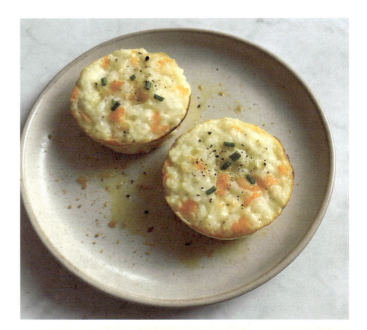

Nutritional Info (per serving)
Calories: ~480 kcal | Protein: ~20 g | Potassium: ~190 mg | Phosphorus: ~95 mg | Sodium: ~160 mg | Fat: ~21 g | Carbs: ~40 g | Cholesterol: 0 mg | Oxalates: ~10 mg

Creativity TWIST:
Try swapping the carrot for mashed zucchini or yellow squash for a milder flavor.

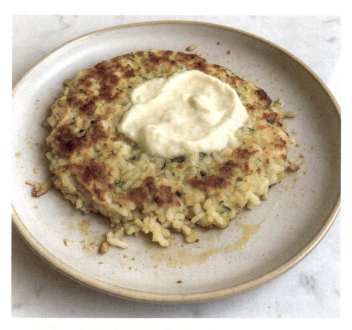

Reno Creamy Rice Frittata

Servings	Prep Time	Cook time	PROTEIN	PHOSPHORUS	SODIUM	POTASSIUM
1	5'	10'	MID	LOW	LOW	LOW

INGREDIENTS
- ½ cup liquid egg whites, low sodium (118 g)
- 3/4 cup cooked white rice (160 g)
- 2 Tbsp peeled zucchini, grated (30 g)
- 1 1/2 Tbsp low-sodium cream cheese (20 g)
- 1 Tbsp olive oil (15 mL) (Pantry)

DIRECTIONS
1. Beat egg whites with rice and zucchini in a bowl.
2. Heat olive oil in skillet, add mixture, cook gently 3–4 minutes.
3. Top with cream cheese, cover, cook 3 more minutes until set.
4. Serve warm.

Nutritional Info (per serving)
Calories: 450 kcal | Protein: 19 g | Potassium: ~350 mg | Phosphorus: ~90 mg | Sodium: ~65 mg | Fat: 19 g | Carbs: 45 g | Cholesterol: 0 mg | Oxalates: 2 mg

Creativity TWIST:
Swap zucchini for shredded peeled apple for a sweet twist.

Canton Banana Breakfast Melt

Servings	Prep Time	Cook time	PROTEIN	PHOSPHORUS	SODIUM	POTASSIUM
1	3'	4'	MID	LOW	LOW	LOW

INGREDIENTS
- 1 slice low-sodium white bread (25 g)
- About 3/4 cup egg whites (160 g)
- 3 oz ripe banana, sliced (40 g)
- 1 1/2 Tbsp honey (25 g) (Pantry)
- 1 Tbsp olive oil (15 mL) (Pantry)

DIRECTIONS
1. Toast bread slice.
2. Scramble egg whites in 1 Tbsp olive oil.
3. Top toast with scrambled egg whites and banana slices.
4. Drizzle honey and remaining olive oil over the to p.
5. Serve warm.

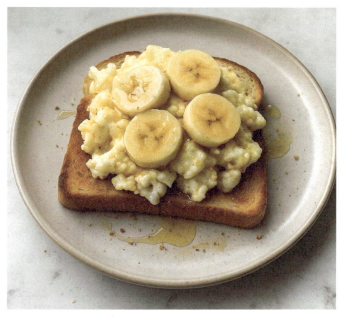

Nutritional Info (per serving)
Calories: 392 kcal | Protein: 19.3 g | Potassium: 395 mg | Phosphorus: 169 mg | Sodium: 259 mg | Fat: 15.8 g | Carbs: 44.7 g | Cholesterol: 0 mg | Oxalates: 4 mg

Creativity TWIST:
Swap honey for maple syrup or try substituting banana with peeled apple slices.

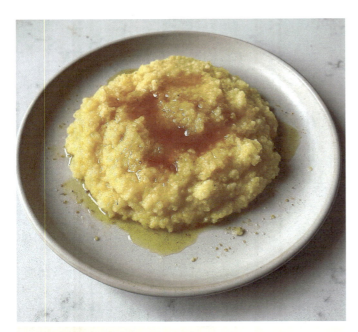

Portland Sunrise Polenta

Servings	Prep Time	Cook time	PROTEIN	PHOSPHORUS	SODIUM	POTASSIUM
1	7'	10'	MID	LOW	LOW	LOW

INGREDIENTS
- 1/3 cup quick-cook polenta (45 g)
- 1/2 cup rice milk (120 mL)
- 1/2 cup egg whites (126 g)
- 1 Tbsp honey (15 g) (Pantry)
- 1 Tbsp olive oil (15 mL) (Pantry)

DIRECTIONS
1. Bring rice milk and 1 Tbsp olive oil to a boil.
2. Whisk in polenta, stirring constantly, then reduce heat to low.
3. Stir in egg whites and cook until mixture thickens and becomes creamy.
4. Serve topped with honey and drizzle remaining olive oil

Nutritional Info (per serving)
Calories: 454 kcal | Protein: 18.0 g | Potassium: 270 mg | Phosphorus: 77 mg | Sodium: 274 mg | Fat: 15.9 g | Carbs: 61 g | Cholesterol: 0 mg | Oxalates: 5 mg

Creativity TWIST:
Add ¼ tsp lemon zest or ground ginger for a fresh, aromatic note

Dayton Apple Oat Cup

Servings	Prep Time	Cook time	PROTEIN	PHOSPHORUS	SODIUM	POTASSIUM
1	5'	5'	MID	LOW	LOW	LOW

INGREDIENTS
- 1/2 cup quick oats (45 g)
- 3/8 cup egg whites (90 g)
- 1/3 cup peeled diced apple (60 g)
- 1 Tbsp honey (21 g) (Pantry)
- 1 Tbsp olive oil (15 mL) (Pantry)

DIRECTIONS
1. Combine oats, apple, and egg whites in a microwave-safe bowl.
2. Microwave on high for 2 minutes, stir, then microwave in 30-second increments until set.
3. Drizzle with honey and olive oil before serving.

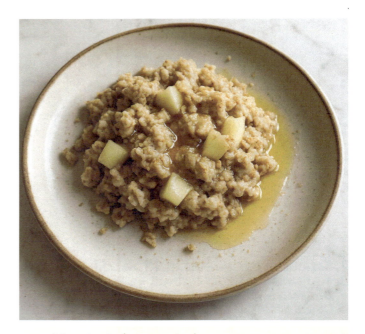

Nutritional Info (per serving)
Calories: 434 kcal | Protein: 16.6 g | Potassium: 373 mg | Phosphorus: 141 mg | Sodium: 169 mg | Fat: 17.5 g | Carbs: 55.3 g | Cholesterol: 0 mg | Oxalates: 11 mg

Creativity TWIST:
Add cinnamon, nutmeg, or top with fresh blueberries for extra flavor and antioxidants.

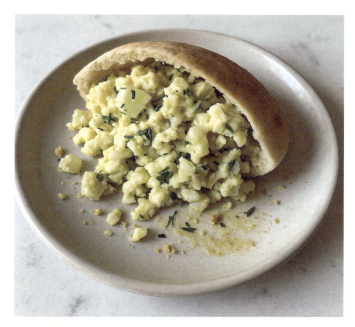

Mobile Mild Egg Salad Pita

Servings	Prep Time	Cook time	PROTEIN	PHOSPHORUS	SODIUM	K POTASSIUM
1	7'	5'	MID	LOW	LOW	LOW

INGREDIENTS
- 1 mini white pita (30 g) (low sodium if available)
- About 2/3 cup egg whites (130 g)
- 2 Tbsp peeled cooked potato, diced (30 g)
- 2 1/4 Tbsp olive oil (34 g) (Pantry)
- Fresh herbs (chives, dill, parsley) for flavor (no salt)

DIRECTIONS
1. Scramble egg whites in 1 Tbsp (about 14 g) olive oil over medium heat.
2. Toss cooked egg whites with diced potato and remaining olive oil.
3. Season with fresh herbs to taste.
4. Fill pita pocket with egg salad mixture and serve immediately.

Nutritional Info (per serving)
Calories: 476 kcal | Protein: 17.4 g | Potassium: 379 mg | Phosphorus: 45 mg | Sodium: 301 mg | Fat: 35 g | Carbs: 23 g | Cholesterol: 0 mg | Oxalates: 7.5 mg

Creativity TWIST:
Try adding a squeeze of lemon juice or a dash of smoked paprika for extra zing.

Salem Peaches & Cream Bowl

Servings	Prep Time	Cook time	PROTEIN	PHOSPHORUS	SODIUM	K POTASSIUM
1	4'	0'	MID	LOW	LOW	LOW

INGREDIENTS
- 2/3 cup low-sodium cottage cheese (150 g)
- 1/4 cup peeled canned peaches, drained (60 g)
- 1/4 cup cooked white rice, cooled (50 g)
- 1 Tbsp honey (21 g) (Pantry)
- 1 Tbsp olive oil (15 mL) (Pantry)

DIRECTIONS
1. Mix cottage cheese, cooked rice, and peaches in a bowl.
2. Drizzle honey and olive oil on to p.
3. Serve immediately and enjoy

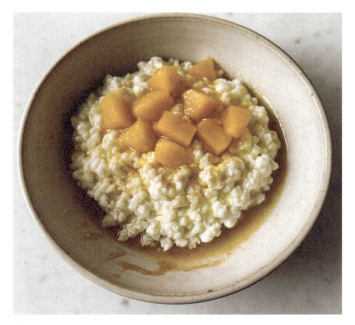

Nutritional Info (per serving)
Calories: 426 kcal | Protein: 18.4 g | Potassium: 275 mg | Phosphorus: 147 mg | Sodium: 107 mg | Fat: 17.7 g | Carbs: 44.4 g | Cholesterol: 15 mg | Oxalates: 10 mg

Creativity TWIST:
Try swapping peaches with pineapple or pears for variety

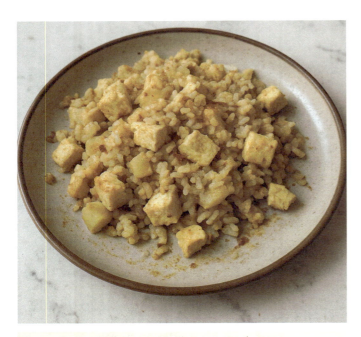

Erie Sunny Tofu Hash

Servings	Prep Time	Cook time	PROTEIN	PHOSPHORUS	SODIUM	POTASSIUM
1	6'	7'	MID	LOW	LOW	LOW

INGREDIENTS
- 3.5 oz firm tofu, drained, pressed, cubed (100 g)
- 1/4 cup peeled cooked potato, diced (40 g)
- 1/4 cup cooked white rice (35 g)
- 1 Tbsp olive oil (15 mL) (Pantry)
- 1 Tbsp mayonnaise (15 g)

DIRECTIONS
1. Sauté tofu and potato in olive oil for 3–4 minutes.
2. Add rice, stir well, cook 2 more minutes.
3. Remove from heat, stir in mayonnaise. Serve warm.

Nutritional Info (per serving)
Calories: 438 kcal | Protein: 17.6 g | Potassium: 272 mg | Phosphorus: 157 mg | Sodium: 98 mg | Fat: 32 g | Carbs: 22.3 g | Cholesterol: 5 mg | Oxalates: 9 mg

Creativity TWIST:
Season with black pepper, or add a sprinkle of fresh basil.

Fresno Sunrise Rice Bowl

Servings	Prep Time	Cook time	PROTEIN	PHOSPHORUS	SODIUM	POTASSIUM
1	4'	0'	MID	LOW	LOW	LOW

INGREDIENTS
- 3/4 cup egg whites (150 g)
- 1/3 cup cooked white rice (75 g)
- 2 Tbsp peeled cooked carrot, finely diced (30 g)
- 1 1/2 Tbsp honey (21 g) (Pantry)
- 1 1/3 Tbsp olive oil (20 mL) (Pantry)

DIRECTIONS
1. Heat rice and carrot in skillet with half the olive oil (10 mL).
2. Pour in egg whites; stir gently until just set.
3. Drizzle with honey and remaining olive oil before serving.

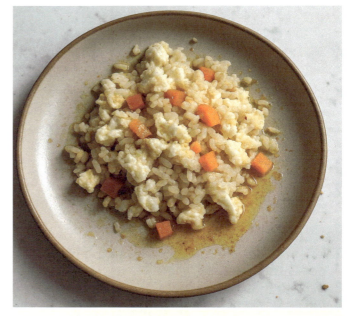

Nutritional Info (per serving)
Calories: 409 kcal | Protein: 18.8 g | Potassium: 346 mg | Phosphorus: 64 mg | Sodium: 292 mg | Fat: 19 g | Carbs: 42 g | Cholesterol: 0 mg | Oxalates: 1.2 mg

Creativity TWIST:
Top with a pinch of cinnamon or fresh chives for added flavor without extra sodium or potassium

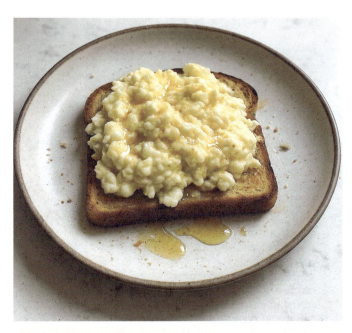

Lincoln Mild Cheese Toast

Servings	Prep Time	Cook time	PROTEIN	PHOSPHORUS	SODIUM	POTASSIUM
1	4'	4'	MID	LOW	LOW	LOW

INGREDIENTS
- 1 slice low-sodium white bread (32 g)
- 3/8 cup egg whites (90 g)
- 3 Tbsp ricotta cheese, whole milk, low sodium (40 g)
- 1 Tbsp olive oil (15 mL) (Pantry)
- 2 Tbsp honey (30 g) (Pantry)

DIRECTIONS
1. Toast the bread.
2. Scramble egg whites with ricotta cheese in a pan with olive oil over medium heat until cooked through.
3. Top toasted bread with the egg and ricotta mixture.
4. Drizzle honey over the top

Nutritional Info (per serving)
Calories: 412 kcal | Protein: 17.2 g | Potassium: 240 mg | Phosphorus: 83 mg | Sodium: 216 mg | Fat: 19.9 g | Carbs: 42.1 g | Cholesterol: 7 mg | Oxalates: 7 mg

CREATIVITY TWIST:
You can swap ricotta for low-sodium cottage cheese for a slightly different texture and taste.

Bismarck Vanilla Rice Bowl

Servings	Prep Time	Cook time	PROTEIN	PHOSPHORUS	SODIUM	POTASSIUM
1	3'	4'	MID	LOW	LOW	LOW

INGREDIENTS
- 1/4 cup cooked white rice (50 g)
- 1/2 cup egg whites (125 g)
- 1/2 cup unsweetened rice milk (120 mL)
- 1 Tbsp honey (21 g) (Pantry)
- 2 Tbsp olive oil (27 g) (Pantry)
- 1/4 tsp vanilla extract (optional)

DIRECTIONS
1. In a small saucepan, gently heat cooked rice, rice milk, and egg whites, stirring constantly until thick and creamy.
2. Remove from heat. Stir in honey, olive oil, and vanilla extract.
3. Serve warm.

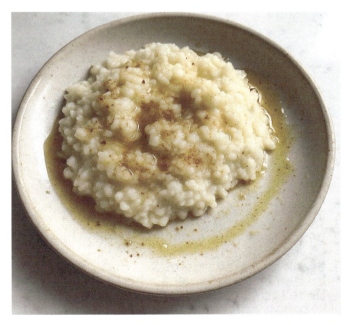

Nutritional Info (per serving)
Calories: 489 kcal | Protein: 15.4 g | Potassium: 277 mg | Phosphorus: 58 mg | Sodium: 269 mg | Fat: 29 g | Carbs: 44 g | Cholesterol: 0 mg | Oxalates: 5 mg

Creativity TWIST:
Top with nutmeg for warm flavor without extra sodium or potassium.

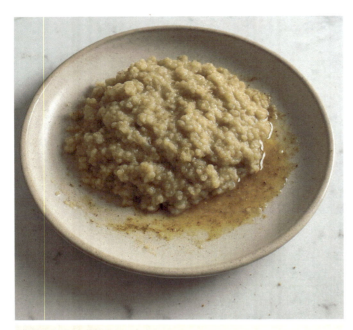

Nutritional Info (per serving)
Calories: 454 kcal | Protein: 18.0 g | Potassium: 270 mg | Phosphorus: 77 mg | Sodium: 274 mg | Fat: 15.9 g | Carbs: 61 g | Cholesterol: 0 mg | Oxalates: 5 mg

Creativity TWIST:
Swap almond milk for coconut milk for a tropical twist

Savannah Olive Scramble

Servings	Prep Time	Cook time	PROTEIN	PHOSPHORUS	SODIUM	POTASSIUM
1	5'	11'	MID	LOW	LOW	LOW

INGREDIENTS
- 2 large eggs (or egg substitute)
- 1 slice white bread (low sodium)
- 2 Tbsp olive oil
- 1 Tbsp chopped parsley (or chives)
- ½ Tbsp unsalted butter (optional)

DIRECTIONS
1. Toast the bread and set aside.
2. Whisk eggs with herbs until fluffy (hand mixer optional).
3. Break up bread into pieces and add to beaten eggs; let soak 1 minute.
4. Heat 1 to 1½ Tbsp olive oil in a pan for 30 seconds. Add egg mixture.
5. Scramble gently while cooking.
6. Drizzle remaining olive oil over toast and eggs before serving.

Trenton Honey Cinnamon Quinoa

Servings	Prep Time	Cook time	PROTEIN	PHOSPHORUS	SODIUM	POTASSIUM
2	5'	20'	MID	LOW	LOW	LOW

INGREDIENTS
- 1/2 cup quinoa, rinsed (80 g)
- 1 cup unsweetened almond milk (240 mL)
- 5 large egg whites (~165 g)
- 1 tsp honey (~7 g) (Pantry)
- 1/4 tsp ground cinnamon (~0.65 g)
- 2 tsp unsalted butter (~9 g)
- 1 tsp extra virgin olive oil (~5 mL) (Pantry)

DIRECTIONS
1. Rinse quinoa well under cold water to remove bitterness.
2. In a small saucepan, combine quinoa and almond milk. Bring to a gentle boil, reduce heat, and simmer covered about 15 minutes until quinoa is tender and liquid mostly absorbed.
3. Meanwhile, lightly whisk egg whites in a small bowl.
4. Remove quinoa from heat; slowly stir in whisked egg whites and cinnamon, mixing quickly to avoid scrambling.
5. Return to very low heat 2–3 minutes, stirring constantly, until mixture thickens like a soft porridge.
6. Remove from heat; stir in honey, unsalted butter, and EVOO. Serve warm.

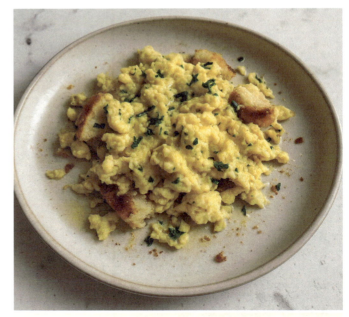

Nutritional Info (per serving)
Calories: 504 kcal | Protein: 15 g | Potassium: 200 mg | Phosphorus: 220 mg | Sodium: 265 mg | Fat: 44 g | Carbs: 14 g | Cholesterol: 388 mg | Oxalates: 5 mg

Creativity TWIST:
Add smoked paprika and lemon zest for flavor; swap parsley for chives or cilantro.

Charleston Cottage Cakes

Servings	Prep Time	Cook time	PROTEIN	PHOSPHORUS	SODIUM	K POTASSIUM
1	5'	10'	MID	LOW	LOW	LOW

INGREDIENTS
- ½ cup (60g) all-purpose flour
- ¼ tsp baking powder (sodium free)
- ½ cup (120 mL) rice milk
- 2 Tbsp (30 mL) olive oil
- 2 Tbsp unsalted butter
- 1 Tbsp maple syrup

DIRECTIONS
1. Mix flour, baking powder, and optional spices in a bowl.
2. Add rice milk and 1 Tbsp olive oil; stir to remove lumps. Don't overmix. Let rest a few minutes. Add more rice milk if too thick.
3. Heat a heavy pan for 1 minute, add 1–1½ Tbsp olive oil.
4. Scoop batter into pan, leaving ½ inch between pancakes. Cook on moderately high heat until bubbles form (1–2 min).
5. Flip carefully, cook 2 more minutes.
6. Add 1–1½ Tbsp olive oil before each new batch.
7. Serve pancakes with butter and syru p.

Nutritional Info (per serving)
Calories: 612 kcal | Protein: 6.7 g | Potassium: 201 mg | Phosphorus: 84 mg | Sodium: 55 mg | Fat: 33.6 g | Carbs: 72.5 g | Cholesterol: 31 mg | Oxalates: ~15 mg

> **Creativity TWIST:** Mix diced apple into the batter. About ¼ cup will be enough.

Maple Grove Egg Plate

Servings	Prep Time	Cook time	PROTEIN	PHOSPHORUS	SODIUM	K POTASSIUM
1	5'	7'	MID	LOW	LOW	LOW

INGREDIENTS
- 2 large eggs
- 2 Tbsp (30 mL) olive oil (total) (pantry)
- 1 Tbsp maple syrup (pantry)
- 1 slice low-sodium white bread
- 1 Tbsp unsalted butter (pantry)

DIRECTIONS
1. Heat skillet on medium for a few minutes.
2. Add 1 Tbsp olive oil and fry egg to your liking.
3. Toast bread with butter.
4. Place toast on plate, top with egg, and drizzle syru p.
5. Add optional toppings for extra flavor.

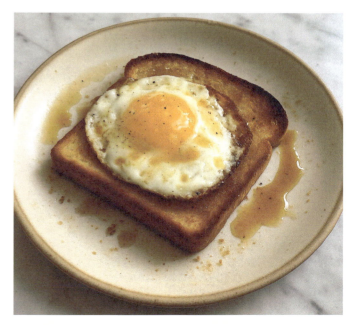

Nutritional Info (per serving)
Calories 599 kcal | Protein 14.6 g | Potassium 231 mg | Phosphorus 219 mg | Sodium 246 mg | Fat 49 g | Carb 26.2 g | Cholesterol 372 mg | Oxalates ~5 mg

> **Creativity TWIST:**
> Serve with 4 baby carrots, ¼ cucumber slices, 2 large strawberries, and 1 rib celery.

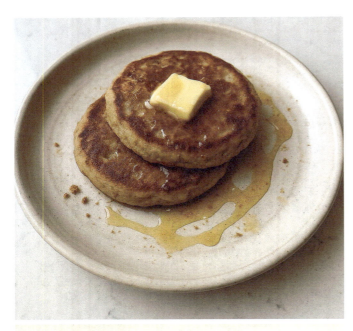

Nutritional Info (per serving)

Calories 423 kcal | Protein 8g | Potassium 110mg | Phosphorus 60mg | Sodium 100mg | Fat 50.5g | Carb 18g | Chol 0mg

Creativity TWIST:
Add cinnamon or ground ginger to the batter

Zagros Berry Cream Bowl

Servings	Prep Time	Cook time	PROTEIN	PHOSPHORUS	SODIUM	POTASSIUM
1	5'	11'	MID	LOW	LOW	LOW

INGREDIENTS
- ½ cup (120g) coconut milk yogurt
- ¼ cup (35g) blueberries
- 1 Tbsp honey (pantry)
- 2 Tbsp rolled oats
- 3 Tbsp (45 mL) olive oil (pantry)

DIRECTIONS
1. In a bowl, add the yogurt, berries, oats, and honey to make one layer.
2. Drizzle 1 Tbsp olive oil over each layer.
3. Then repeat the process two times.
4. Dig in and enjoy!

Albany Almond Pancakes

Servings	Prep Time	Cook time	PROTEIN	PHOSPHORUS	SODIUM	POTASSIUM
2	10'	10'	LOW	LOW	LOW	LOW

INGREDIENTS
- ½ cup (60g) flour
- 1 Tbsp almond butter
- 1 tsp almond extract
- 1 large egg, beaten
- ¼ cup (60 mL) rice milk
- ½ teaspoon baking powder (pantry)
- 3 Tbsp (45 mL) olive oil (total) – (pantry)
- 1 Tbsp unsalted butter (pantry)
- 1 Tbsp honey (pantry)

DIRECTIONS
1. Mix flour and baking powder in a small bowl.
2. In another bowl, combine almond butter, almond extract, rice milk, beaten egg, and 1 Tbsp olive oil. Add 2 Tbsp rice milk if batter is too thick.
3. Add liquid to flour and mix until moistened. Don't overbeat.
4. Heat 2 Tbsp oil in a large skillet over medium heat for 2 minutes.
5. Scoop ¼ cup batter into skillet, keeping pancakes separate. Cook 2 minutes until bubbles form.
6. Flip and cook another 2 minutes. Remove from heat.
7. Stack pancakes, top with 1 Tbsp butter, and drizzle honey.

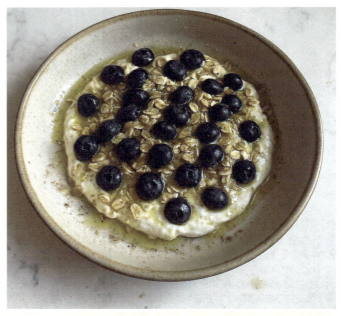

Nutritional Info (per serving)

Calories 677 kcal | Protein 4g | Potassium 190mg | Phosphorus 95mg | Sodium 45mg | Fat 56.5g | Carb 36g | Chol 0mg| Oxalates: 13mg

Creativity TWIST:
Top with a sprig of mint or peeled pear slices.

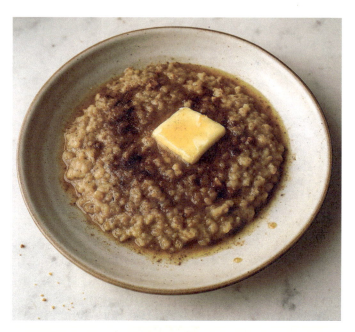

Burlington Cinnamon Oats

Servings	Prep Time	Cook time	PROTEIN	PHOSPHORUS	SODIUM	POTASSIUM
1	5'	5'	LOW	LOW	LOW	LOW

INGREDIENTS
- ⅓ cup instant oats (30 g)
- ⅔ cup water (160 mL) (Pantry)
- ½ tsp cinnamon (Pantry)
- 2 Tbsp olive oil (30 mL) (Pantry)
- 2 Tbsp unsalted butter (28 g) (Pantry)
- 1 Tbsp honey (20 mL) (Pantry)

DIRECTIONS
1. In a small pot, boil water with olive oil.
2. Add oats, cinnamon, and honey. Stir.
3. Simmer on low heat until mixture boils gently.
4. Remove from heat and pour directly into a breakfast cereal bowl.
5. Add butter on top of oatmeal for extra flavor and calories.

Nutritional Info (per serving)
Calories 607 kcal | Protein 4g | Potassium 140mg | Phosphorus 90mg | Sodium 100mg | Fat 52.5g | Carb 42g | Chol 0mg

Creativity TWIST:
Add ¼ cup peeled, diced apple or ½ tsp vanilla extract for flavor depth.

Sonoma Soft Wrap Morning

Servings	Prep Time	Cook time	PROTEIN	PHOSPHORUS	SODIUM	POTASSIUM
1	5'	5'	LOW	LOW	LOW	LOW

INGREDIENTS
- small white flour tortilla
- 1 large egg
- 3 Tbsp (45 mL) olive oil (total) (pantry)
- 1 Tbsp butter (pantry)
- 1 Tbsp shredded lettuce (optional)
- 1 tsp mild salsa (low-sodium) (pantry)

DIRECTIONS
1. Heat 1 Tbsp oil in a small pan for 30 seconds.
2. Cook tortilla 1 minute per side.
3. Remove tortilla, brush with butter.
4. Heat 1 Tbsp olive oil in another pan on medium-high for 30 seconds.
5. Add egg and scramble until cooked.
6. Add egg, salsa, and lettuce to tortilla.
7. Drizzle with 1 Tbsp extra virgin olive oil before serving.

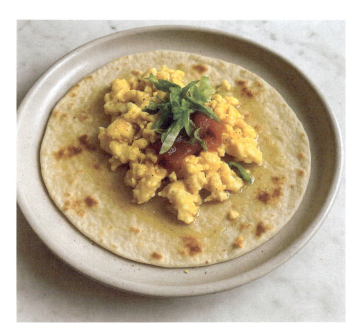

Nutritional Info (per serving)
Calories 677 kcal | Protein 10g | Potassium 190mg | Phosphorus 110mg | Sodium 235mg | Fat 62.5g | Carb 16g | Chol 180mg

Creativity TWIST:
Add 2 large cooked shrimp pieces to the tortilla along with the egg, lettuce, and salsa

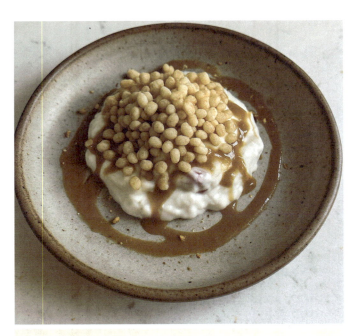

Coral Bay Crunch Cup

Servings	Prep Time	Cook time	PROTEIN	PHOSPHORUS	SODIUM	POTASSIUM
1	7'	0'	LOW	LOW	LOW	LOW

INGREDIENTS
- ¼ cup (15g) unsweetened rice puffs
- ¼ cup (60g) coconut yogurt
- 1 Tbsp sunflower seed butter
- 1 Tbsp honey (pantry)
- 2 Tbsp (30 mL) olive oil (pantry)

DIRECTIONS
1. In a small bowl, mix 1 Tbsp sunflower seed butter with 2 Tbsp olive oil and 1 Tbsp honey. Set aside.
2. In a medium-sized bowl, layer the rice puffs, yogurt, and optional diced strawberry.Then drizzle the layer with the sunflower butter mixture.
3. Continue adding other layers until all ingredients are used u p.

Nutritional Info (per serving)
Calories 567 kcal | Protein 5g | Potassium 150mg | Phosphorus 85mg | Sodium 50mg | Fat 41.5g | Carb 30g | Chol 0mg

Creativity TWIST:
(Optional but recommended) Add 2 diced large strawberries for a little gourmet flavor.

Lexington Light Bagel Stack

Servings	Prep Time	Cook time	PROTEIN	PHOSPHORUS	SODIUM	POTASSIUM
1	5'	2'	LOW	LOW	LOW	LOW

INGREDIENTS
- ½ mini plain bagel (low sodium) (about 40 g)
- 2 Tbsp whipped cream cheese (low sodium) (30 mL / approx. 28 g)
- 2 slices peeled cucumber (about 20 g)
- 1 slice roasted red pepper (about 15 g)
- 2 Tbsp olive oil (30 mL) (Pantry)
- ¼ tsp black pepper (Pantry)

DIRECTIONS
1. Toast the bagel and spread whipped cream cheese evenly on to p.
2. Layer cucumber slices and roasted red pepper on the bagel.
3. Drizzle with olive oil and sprinkle black pepper before serving.

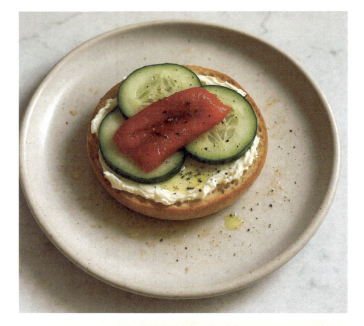

Nutritional Info (per serving)
Calories: 488 kcal | Protein: 6 g | Potassium: 240 mg | Phosphorus: 85 mg | Sodium: 195 mg | Fat: 40.5 g | Carbs: 20 g | Cholesterol: 15 mg

CREATIVITY TWIST:
For a bit of crunch, add toasted pine nuts or finely chopped radishes on to p.

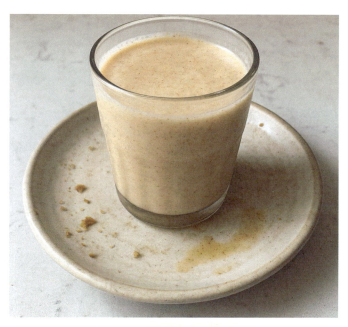

Route 66 Sunrise Smoothie

Servings	Prep Time	Cook time	PROTEIN	PHOSPHORUS	SODIUM	POTASSIUM
1	5'	0'	MID	LOW	MID	LOW

INGREDIENTS
- ½ cup (120 mL) rice milk
- ¼ cup (40 g) peeled frozen pear slices
- 2 Tbsp (30 mL) olive oil (unsalted) (Pantry)
- 1 Tbsp honey (Pantry)
- 3 large egg whites (~100 g)
- Dash cinnamon (Pantry)

DIRECTIONS
1. Blend all ingredients until smooth.
2. Serve chilled.

Nutritional Info (per serving)
Calories: 437 kcal | Protein: 11.4 g | Potassium: 276 mg | Phosphorus: 42 mg | Sodium: 202 mg | Fat: 29.7 g | Carbs: 33.7 g | Cholesterol: 0 mg | Oxalates: N/A

Creativity TWIST:
Add fresh mint or a splash of lemon juice for extra freshness.

Backyard Strawberry Shortshake

Servings	Prep Time	Cook time	PROTEIN	PHOSPHORUS	SODIUM	POTASSIUM
1	7'	0'	LOW	LOW	LOW	LOW

INGREDIENTS
- 1 cup (150 g) frozen strawberries
- ¼ medium ripe banana (30 g)
- ½ cup (120 mL) unsweetened almond milk (low sodium preferred)
- 6 Tbsp plain low-fat Greek yogurt
- 2 large egg whites
- 2 Tbsp (30 mL) extra-virgin olive oil (Pantry)
- 1 tsp honey (Pantry)

DIRECTIONS
1. Add strawberries, banana, almond milk, Greek yogurt, egg whites, and olive oil to the blender.
2. Blend until smooth, scraping down sides as needed.
3. Taste; drizzle in honey and pulse once more. Serve chilled.

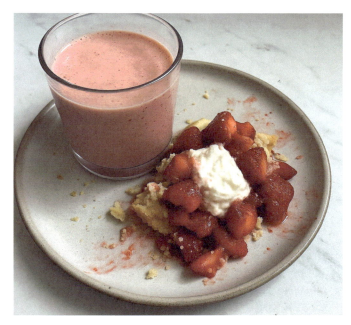

Nutritional Info (per serving)
Calories: ~560 kcal | Protein: ~19 g | Potassium: ~370 mg | Phosphorus: ~180 mg | Sodium: ~130 mg | Fat: ~28 g | Carbs: ~28 g | Cholesterol: ~10 mg | Oxalates: ~8 mg

Creativity TWIST:
Add fresh mint or vanilla extract for a fresh flavor boost.

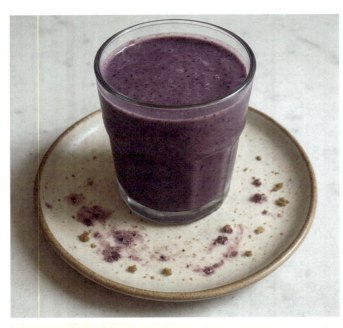

Abyss Blueberry Bliss

Servings	Prep Time	Cook time	PROTEIN	PHOSPHORUS	SODIUM	POTASSIUM
1	5'	0'	MID	LOW	MID	LOW

INGREDIENTS
- ¾ cup (110 g) frozen blueberries
- ½ cup (120 mL) unsweetened almond milk
- 4 large egg whites
- 1 Tbsp quick oats
- 2 Tbsp (30 mL) extra-virgin olive oil (Pantry)
- 1 tsp honey (Pantry)

DIRECTIONS
1. Blend blueberries, almond milk, egg whites, oats, and olive oil until creamy.
2. Sweeten with honey, pulse briefly, and pour into a chilled glass.

Nutritional Info (per serving)
Calories: 439 kcal | Protein: 16.4 g | Potassium: 209 mg | Phosphorus: 92 mg | Sodium: 247 mg | Fat: 29.3 g | Carbs: 28.8 g | Cholesterol: 0 mg | Oxalates: ~17 mg

Creativity TWIST:
Add a drop of pure vanilla extract and a curl of lemon zest for a New England-inspired flavor.

Sunset Peach-Pine Splash

Servings	Prep Time	Cook time	PROTEIN	PHOSPHORUS	SODIUM	POTASSIUM
1	5	0'	LOW	LOW	LOW	LOW

INGREDIENTS
- ⅓ cup (80 g) canned peaches, juice-packed, drained
- ⅓ cup (50 g) frozen pineapple chunks
- ½ cup (120 mL) unsweetened almond milk
- 7 Tbsp (105 g) plain low-fat Greek yogurt
- 3 Tbsp (45 mL) extra-virgin olive oil (Pantry)
- 1 tsp honey (Pantry)

DIRECTIONS
1. Blend peaches, pineapple, almond milk, Greek yogurt, and olive oil until silky.
2. Add honey, pulse once, and serve over crushed ice if desired.

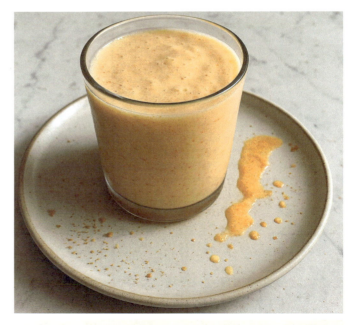

Nutritional Info (per serving)
Calories: ~544 kcal | Protein: ~14.3 g | Potassium: ~370 mg | Phosphorus: ~145 mg | Sodium: ~230 mg | Fat: ~44 g | Carbs: ~30 g | Cholesterol: ~7 mg | Oxalates: ~2 mg

Creativity TWIST:
Add a splash of fresh lime juice or a few fresh mint leaves to brighten the tropical flavors

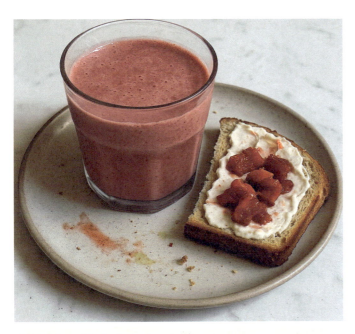

Lato Cranberry Cooler

Servings	Prep Time	Cook time	PROTEIN	PHOSPHORUS	SODIUM	POTASSIUM
1	5'	0'	MID	LOW	MID	LOW

INGREDIENTS
- ½ cup (120 mL) unsweetened cranberry juice
- ½ cup (75 g) frozen strawberries
- ⅓ cup (80 mL) unsweetened almond milk (low sodium)
- 7 Tbsp plain low-fat Greek yogurt
- 3 Tbsp (45 mL) extra-virgin olive oil (Pantry)
- 1 tsp honey (Pantry)

DIRECTIONS
1. Pour cranberry juice, strawberries, almond milk, Greek yogurt, and olive oil into a blender.
2. Blend until smooth and frothy.
3. Stir in honey to taste and enjoy immediately.

Nutritional Info (per serving)
Calories: 591 kcal | Protein: 11.8 g | Potassium: 365 mg | Phosphorus: 226 mg | Sodium: 186 mg | Fat: 47.4 g | Carbs: 33.2 g | Cholesterol: 10 mg | Oxalates: ~5 mg

Creativity TWIST:
Add a pinch of freshly grated ginger for a zingy kick.

Golden Fields Apple Pie Smoothie

Servings	Prep Time	Cook time	PROTEIN	PHOSPHORUS	SODIUM	POTASSIUM
1	7'	0'	LOW	LOW	LOW	LOW

INGREDIENTS
- ¾ cup (210 g) unsweetened applesauce
- 1 Tbsp quick oats
- ½ cup (120 mL) unsweetened low-sodium almond milk
- 4 Tbsp plain low-fat Greek yogurt
- 2½ Tbsp (37.5 mL) extra-virgin olive oil (Pantry)
- ¼ tsp ground cinnamon (Pantry)

DIRECTIONS
1. Place applesauce, oats, almond milk, Greek yogurt, and olive oil in a blender.
2. Blitz until perfectly smooth.
3. Sprinkle in cinnamon, pulse once, and pour into your favorite mug.

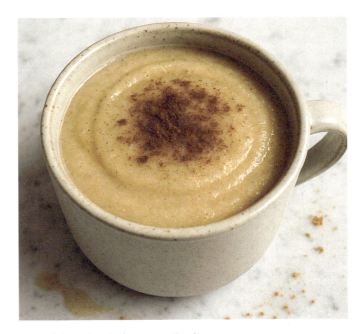

Nutritional Info (per serving)
Calories: ~520 kcal | Protein: ~10 g | Potassium: ~210 mg | Phosphorus: ~80 mg | Sodium: ~130 mg | Fat: ~38 g | Carbs: ~27 g | Cholesterol: ~6 mg | Oxalates: ~11 mg

Creativity TWIST:
For a caramel apple twist, drizzle ½ tsp honey in the glass before pouring to create a sweet ribbon

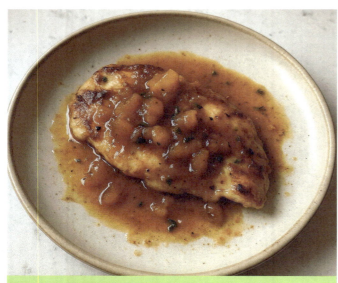

Recommended Side Dish
Herbed Golden Couscous p. 50 (Soaks up the glaze)

Nutritional Info (per serving)
Calories: ~510 kcal | Protein: 26 g | Potassium: 379 mg | Phosphorus: 209 mg | Sodium: 64 mg | Fat: 21.4 g | Carbs: 21.6 g | Cholesterol: 81 mg | Oxalates: <50 mg

Shiraz Peach-Glazed Chicken Cutlets

Servings	Prep Time	Cook time	PROTEIN	PHOSPHORUS	SODIUM	POTASSIUM
1	8'	12'	MID	LOW	MID	LOW

INGREDIENTS
- 4 oz (113 g) chicken breast, sliced thinly as a cutlet
- ¼ cup (60 g) no-salt canned peach slices, diced
- 1 Tbsp (20 g) low-sugar peach preserves
- 3 Tbsp (42 g) unsalted butter (pantry)
- 1 tsp fresh thyme leaves

DIRECTIONS
1. Pat chicken dry, season with pepper and thyme.
2. Heat 2 tbsp butter over medium-high heat; sear chicken 3 minutes per side.
3. Stir in peach preserves and 2 tbsp water; simmer 2 minutes until glossy. Remove chicken, keep warm.
4. Add 1 tbsp butter to glaze, stir until combined. Spoon over chicken and serve.

Creativity TWIST:
Serve over a bed of lightly sautéed spinach or baby arugula for a fresh, peppery contrast.

Sir James Rosemary Turkey

Servings	Prep Time	Cook time	PROTEIN	PHOSPHORUS	SODIUM	POTASSIUM
1	7'	13'	MID	LOW	LOW	LOW

INGREDIENTS
- 4 oz (113 g) turkey tenderloin, raw, sliced ½-inch thick
- 2 Tbsp (30 g) seedless red grapes, halved
- 1 Tbsp (15 ml) dry white wine (or low-sodium broth)
- 3 Tbsp (42 g) extra-virgin olive oil (pantry)
- 1 sprig fresh rosemary

DIRECTIONS
1. Heat olive oil 1 min over medium heat. Brown turkey and rosemary, 2 min per medallion side.
2. Add grapes and wine; cover pan with lid and simmer on low heat, 6 min until turkey hits 165°F (74 celcius).
3. Simmer 1 min more to reduce sauce.
4. Serve turkey topped with grapes.

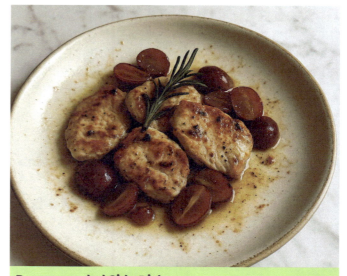

Recommended Side Dish
Leached Garlic Mashed Potatoes, p. 69 (Classic Pair)

Nutritional Info (per serving)
Calories: 504 kcal | Protein: 25.6 g | Potassium: 320 mg | Phosphorus: 197 mg | Sodium: 44 mg | Fat: 42.1 g | Carbs: 3.8 g | Cholesterol: 72 mg | Oxalates: <5 mg

Creativity TWIST:
Try sliced pears instead of grapes for autumn flair or add a pinch of fresh thyme alongside rosemary.

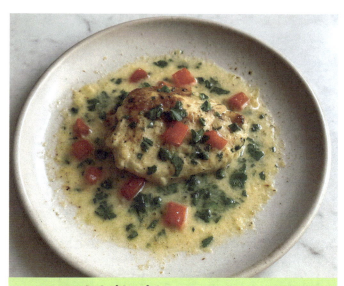

Recommended Side Dish
Lemon-Parsley White Rice (Tropical match), p. 68

Nutritional Info (per serving)
Calories: 545 kcal | Protein: 18 g | Potassium: 332 mg | Phosphorus: 161 mg | Sodium: 64 mg | Fat: 53 g | Carbs: 4 g | Cholesterol: 94 mg | Oxalates: <50 mg

Key West Lime-Coconut Chicken

Servings	Prep Time	Cook time	PROTEIN	PHOSPHORUS	SODIUM	POTASSIUM
1	10'	15'	MID	LOW	MID	LOW

INGREDIENTS
- 3 oz (85 g) chicken thigh, skin removed
- ¼ cup (60 ml) lite canned coconut milk
- 1 Tbsp (15 ml) fresh lime juice with zest
- 2 Tbsp (30 g) diced mild red bell pepper
- 1 Tbsp (5 g) chopped cilantro
- 2 Tbsp (28 ml) olive oil (pantry)

DIRECTIONS
1. Heat olive oil in a small frying pan.
2. Sauté chicken for 4 minutes on medium-high heat.
3. Add red bell pepper; cook 3 more minutes.
4. Pour coconut milk and lime juice into pan; simmer on low heat 6 minutes until thickened.
5. Finish with chopped cilantro

Creativity TWIST:
Add a pinch of smoked paprika or cumin for a subtle smoky warmth.

Maple Grove Dijon Chicken Tenders

Servings	Prep Time	Cook time	PROTEIN	PHOSPHORUS	SODIUM	POTASSIUM
1	5	12'	MID	LOW	LOW	LOW

INGREDIENTS
- 2.6 oz (75 g) chicken breast strips, uncooked
- 1 Tbsp (20 g) pure maple syrup (pantry)
- 1 tsp (5 g) Dijon mustard (low-sodium)
- ½ cup (60 g) sliced zucchini rounds
- 2 Tbsp (28 ml) olive oil (pantry)

DIRECTIONS
1. In a bowl, combine chicken, maple syrup, and Dijon mustard; coat thoroughly.
2. Heat olive oil in skillet over medium heat for 1 minute.
3. Sear chicken 3 minutes on high heat.
4. Add zucchini; cook 5 more minutes.
5. Pour remaining glaze over chicken; cook 2 minutes on medium-high heat until sticky.
6. Serve immediately.

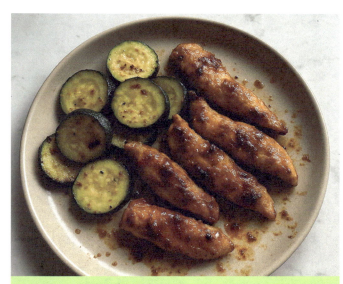

Recommended Side Dish
Honey-Dill Glazed Carrots (Sweet/Savory), p. 73

Nutritional Info (per serving)
Calories: 395 kcal | Protein: 17.9 g | Potassium: 386 mg | Phosphorus: 170 mg | Sodium: 104 mg | Fat: 29.4 g | Carbs: 15.7 g | Cholesterol: 42 mg | Oxalates: 4 mg

Creativity TWIST:
Swap zucchini for thin apple wedges for sweet-savory crunch or sprinkle fresh thyme.

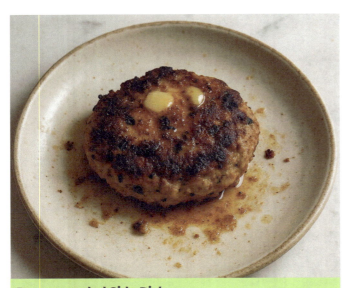

Recommended Side Dish
Roasted Turnip "Fries" (Burger & Fry vibes)

Nutritional Info (per serving)
Calories: 363 kcal | Protein: 23 g | Potassium: 301 mg |
Phosphorus: 229 mg | Sodium: 53 mg | Fat: 27 g | Carbs:
12 g | Cholesterol: 80 mg | Oxalates: 12 mg

Nashville Honey-Herb Turkey Patties

Servings	Prep Time	Cook time	PROTEIN	PHOSPHORUS	SODIUM	POTASSIUM
1	8'	10'	MID	LOW	MID	LOW

INGREDIENTS
- 3.5 oz (100 g) 93% lean ground turkey
- 1 Tbsp (9 g) rolled oats (binder)
- ½ tsp (2 g) honey, warmed (pantry)
- ¼ tsp (1 g) smoked paprika
- 1 tsp (1 g) chopped parsley
- 2 tsp (10 ml) olive oil (pantry)
- 1 Tbsp (14 g) unsalted butter (pantry)

DIRECTIONS
1. Mix turkey, oats, paprika, and parsley in bowl.
2. Form one ¾-inch (2 cm) patty.
3. Heat olive oil in pan over medium-high heat; pan-sear patty 4 minutes per side.
4. Brush warmed honey on patty during last 30 seconds of cooking.
5. After cooking, add unsalted butter on top to melt.

Creativity TWIST:
Serve on a small corn tortilla with shredded lettuce (~55 kcal), add lime squeeze for zestiness.

Catalina Citrus Chicken & Peppers

Servings	Prep Time	Cook time	PROTEIN	PHOSPHORUS	SODIUM	POTASSIUM
1	9'	14'	MID	LOW	LOW	LOW

INGREDIENTS
- 2.5 oz (71 g) chicken breast, cut in chunks
- ½ cup (120 g) canned low-potassium mandarin oranges, rinsed
- ¼ cup (30 g) green bell pepper, julienned
- 1 tsp light soy substitute sauce (15 mg sodium)
- 1 Tbsp (15 ml) olive oil (pantry)
- 1 Tbsp (14 g) unsalted butter (pantry)

DIRECTIONS
1. Stir-fry chicken and bell pepper in olive oil for 5–7 minutes in medium skillet.
2. Add mandarins and soy substitute sauce; cook 3 minutes until glazed.
3. Remove from heat; stir in unsalted butter until melted.
4. Serve warm over lettuce leaves if desired.

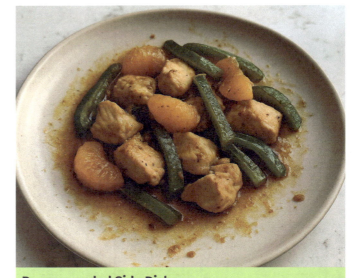

Recommended Side Dish
Garlic-Infused Penne (Pasta cuts the acidity)

Nutritional Info (per serving)
Calories: 398 kcal | Protein: 23 g | Potassium: 295 mg
| Phosphorus: 165 mg | Sodium: 76 mg | Fat: 27.5 g |
Carbs: 15.5 g | Cholesterol: 53 mg | Oxalates: <50 mg

Creativity TWIST:
Add a few fresh basil leaves or a sprinkle of dried oregano for Mediterranean notes.

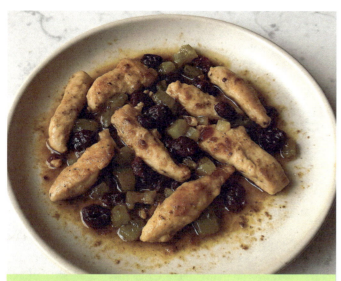

Recommended Side Dish
Herbed Golden Couscous (Holiday flavors)

Nutritional Info (per serving)
Calories: 371 kcal | Protein: 21.3 g | Potassium: 340 mg | Phosphorus: 195 mg | Sodium: 199 mg | Fat: 25 g | Carbs: 16 g | Cholesterol: 78 mg | Oxalates: 12 mg

Verona Cranberry Chicken Sauté

Servings	Prep Time	Cook time	PROTEIN	PHOSPHORUS	SODIUM	K POTASSIUM
1	6'	13'	MID	LOW	MID	LOW

INGREDIENTS
- 3.5 oz (99 g) chicken thighs, cut into strips
- 2 Tbsp (20 g) dried cranberries, reduced-sugar
- ¼ cup (60 ml) low-sodium chicken broth
- ¼ cup (40 g) diced celery (softened)
- 1 tsp (2.3 g) Italian seasoning (dried herbs blend, salt-free)
- 1 Tbsp (13.5 ml) olive oil (pantry)

DIRECTIONS
1. Heat olive oil in skillet; sauté chicken strips 4 minutes on medium-high heat.
2. Add celery and Italian seasoning; cook 3 more minutes.
3. Add broth; stir in cranberries. Simmer on low heat 4 minutes until glossy.

Creativity TWIST:
Add garlic powder or smoked paprika with Italian seasoning for smoky, savory flavor

Santa Fe Chili-Lime Turkey Strips

Servings	Prep Time	Cook time	PROTEIN	PHOSPHORUS	SODIUM	K POTASSIUM
1	7'	10'	MID	LOW	LOW	LOW

INGREDIENTS
- 3 oz (85 g) turkey breast, cut into small strips
- ¼ cup (60 g) canned low-sodium diced tomatoes, drained
- 1 Tbsp (15 ml) lime juice (pantry)
- ¼ tsp mild chili powder (pantry)
- 2.5 tsp (12 g) olive oil (pantry)
- 2.5 Tbsp (35 g) unsalted butter (pantry)

DIRECTIONS
1. Coat turkey strips in chili powder.
2. Heat 1.5 tsp olive oil in skillet; stir-fry turkey 4 minutes. Add tomatoes and lime juice; cook 4 minutes.
3. Keep cooking to Reduce liquid 2 minutes to glaze. Remove the mixture and set aside.
4. Melt butter with 1 tsp olive oil; toss turkey to coat evenly. Serve warm.

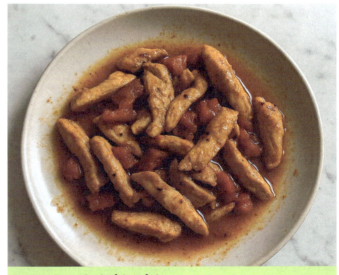

Recommended Side Dish
Zucchini & Corn Sauté (Southwest style)

Nutritional Info (per serving)
Calories: 482 kcal | Protein: 20 g | Potassium: 372 mg | Phosphorus: 177 mg | Sodium: 130 mg | Fat: 39 g | Carbs: 4 g | Cholesterol: 52 mg | Oxalates: <50 mg

Creativity TWIST:
Top with 1 Tbsp diced avocado for creaminess (+55 mg potassium).

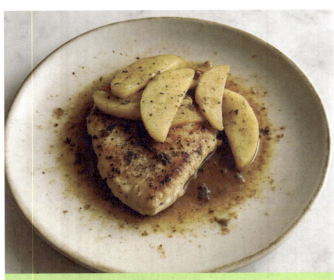

Recommended Side Dish
Leached Garlic Mashed Potatoes (Comfort food)

Nutritional Info (per serving)
Calories: 449 kcal | Protein: 20.4 g | Potassium: 282 mg
| Phosphorus: 135 mg | Sodium: 49 mg | Fat: 38.4 g |
Carbs: 9.7 g | Cholesterol: 141 mg | Oxalates: ~13 mg

Creativity TWIST:
Replace sage with rosemary; apple with pear for winter warmth

Blue Ridge Apple-Sage Chicken

Servings	Prep Time	Cook time	PROTEIN	PHOSPHORUS	SODIUM	POTASSIUM
1	8'	14'	MID	LOW	MID	LOW

INGREDIENTS
- 2.25 oz (64 g) chicken breast tenders
- ½ cup (60 g) peeled sweet apple, thinly sliced
- 1 Tbsp (15 ml) apple cider (or water) (pantry)
- 3 Tbsp (42 g) unsalted butter (pantry)
- ½ tsp dried sage (spice)

DIRECTIONS
1. Melt butter in small skillet.
2. Brown chicken in butter 3 minutes per side.
3. Add apples, cider, and sage. Cover; let apples soften 6 minutes.
4. Uncover; cook on low until sauce reduces (~2 minutes).

Tomato-Basil Chicken Piccata

Servings	Prep Time	Cook time	PROTEIN	PHOSPHORUS	SODIUM	POTASSIUM
1	9'	12'	MID	LOW	LOW	LOW

INGREDIENTS
- 2.5 oz (71 g) chicken breast, pounded
- 2 Tbsp (20 g) halved cherry tomatoes
- 1 Tbsp (15 ml) lemon juice (pantry)
- 3 Tbsp (42 g) unsalted butter (pantry)
- 1 Tbsp (2 g) fresh basil, cut in ribbons

DIRECTIONS
1. Sear chicken in butter 3 minutes per side in small skillet.
2. Add tomatoes and lemon juice; simmer 4 minutes.
3. Top with basil; cover and rest 3 minutes.
4. Spoon sauce over chicken and serve.

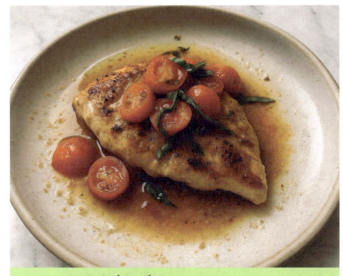

Recommended Side Dish
Garlic-Infused Penne (Italian classic)

Nutritional Info (per serving)
Calories: 426 kcal | Protein: 23 g | Potassium: 333 mg |
Phosphorus: 180 mg | Sodium: 47 mg | Fat: 38 g | Carbs:
2.5 g | Cholesterol: 147 mg | Oxalates: ~20 mg

Creativity TWIST:
Add ¼ tsp capers if sodium budget allows. Swap butter for EVOO to increase healthy fats.

Viennese Velvet Beef Strips

Servings	Prep Time	Cook time	PROTEIN	PHOSPHORUS	SODIUM	POTASSIUM
2	10'	15'	MID	LOW	MID	LOW

INGREDIENTS
- 150 g beef sirloin, thinly sliced
- 50 g tomato, diced
- ½ small onion (75 g), thinly sliced
- 3 Tbsp (40.5 g) olive oil (pantry)
- 2 Tbsp (28 g) unsalted butter (pantry)
- 1 tsp dried thyme (or fresh)

DIRECTIONS
1. Heat 2 Tbsp olive oil and 2 Tbsp butter in skillet over medium heat 1 minute.
2. Add onion; sauté until translucent (~3 minutes).
3. Add beef; stir-fry 4–5 minutes until browned.
4. Add tomato and thyme; simmer 3 minutes.
5. Stir in remaining 1 Tbsp olive oil.
6. Season with pepper and salt substitute to taste. Serve immediately.

Recommended Side Dish
Garlic-Infused Penne (Stroganoff style)

Nutritional Info (per serving)
Calories: 450 kcal | Protein: 17 g | Potassium: 382 mg | Phosphorus: 146 mg | Sodium: 27 mg | Fat: 42 g | Carbs: 5 g | Cholesterol: 58 mg | Oxalates: 2 mg

Creativity TWIST:
Stir in a splash of red wine or balsamic vinegar toward the end of cooking for richness.

Nord Beef, Zucchini Sauté & Fried Egg

Servings	Prep Time	Cook time	PROTEIN	PHOSPHORUS	SODIUM	POTASSIUM
2	8'	12'	MID	LOW	LOW	MID

INGREDIENTS
- 250 g lean flank steak, thinly sliced
- 100 g zucchini, sliced in half-moons
- 1 clove garlic, minced
- 1 Tbsp (15 ml) olive oil (pantry)
- 1 Tbsp (14 g) unsalted butter (pantry)
- 2 large eggs
- 1 tsp dried Italian herb blend (pantry)

DIRECTIONS
1. Toss steak with Italian herbs and pepper.
2. Heat olive oil; sauté garlic 30 seconds.
3. Add steak; stir-fry 3–4 minutes until browned. Remove and keep warm.
4. Sauté zucchini 5 minutes until tender. Return steak; stir 2 minutes.
5. Wipe pan; melt butter; fry eggs sunny-side up (~3 minutes).
6. Serve beef mixture topped with eggs; season eggs with pepper and salt substitute.

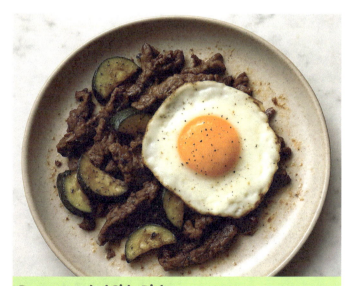

Recommended Side Dish
Roasted Turnip "Fries" (Adds starch to the veg)

Nutritional Info (per serving)
Calories: 370 kcal | Protein: 30 g | Potassium: 517 mg | Phosphorus: 154 mg | Sodium: 54 mg | Fat: 26 g | Carbs: 1.3 g | Cholesterol: 126 mg | Oxalates: 1.5 mg

Creativity TWIST:
For a spicy kick, sprinkle red pepper flakes on the eggs or stir in chopped sun-dried tomatoes.

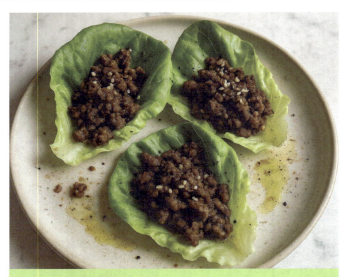

Recommended Side Dish
Asian-Style Sesame-Scallion Rice (Completes the bowl)

Nutritional Info (per serving)
Calories: 383 kcal | Protein: 17.4 g | Potassium: 365 mg | Phosphorus: 142 mg | Sodium: 289 mg | Fat: 36 g | Carbs: 4 g | Cholesterol: 48

Tokyo Beef Lettuce Cups

Servings	Prep Time	Cook time	PROTEIN	PHOSPHORUS	SODIUM	POTASSIUM
2	10'	10'	MID	LOW	LOW	LOW

INGREDIENTS
- 120 g lean ground beef
- 2 tsp (10 ml) low-sodium soy sauce (or tamari)
- 1 tsp (5 g) grated ginger
- 8 large butter lettuce leaves
- 4 Tbsp (60 ml) extra virgin olive oil (pantry)

DIRECTIONS
1. Heat 2 Tbsp EVOO in skillet over medium heat 1 minute.
2. Add beef and ginger; cook 5 minutes until browned.
3. Stir in soy sauce; cook 2 more minutes; remove from heat.
4. Spoon beef mixture into lettuce leaves.
5. Drizzle remaining 2 Tbsp EVOO over filled cups.
6. Season with pepper and optional sesame seeds. Roll and serve immediately.

Creativity TWIST:
Add finely chopped water chestnuts or toasted sesame seeds for crunch.

Oklahoma Comfort Ginger-Beef

Servings	Prep Time	Cook time	PROTEIN	PHOSPHORUS	SODIUM	POTASSIUM
2	8'	15'	MID	LOW	LOW	LOW

INGREDIENTS
- 120 g lean ground beef
- 1 cup (150 g) cooked white rice
- 1 tsp minced ginger
- 1 Tbsp (15 ml) olive oil (pantry)
- 1 tsp rice vinegar (pantry)
- 2 large eggs

DIRECTIONS
1. Warm rice; divide between two bowls.
2. Heat olive oil in skillet; sauté ginger 30 seconds. Add beef; cook 5 minutes until browned.
3. Stir in vinegar; cook 1 minute.
4. Spoon beef over rice.
5. Fry eggs sunny-side up (~3 minutes); place atop bowls.
6. Season with pepper and salt substitute.

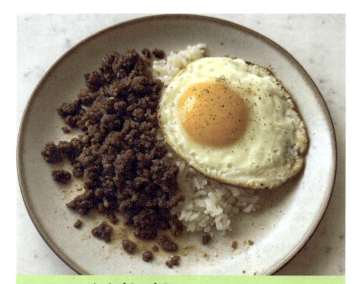

Recommended Side Dish
Asian-Style Sesame-Scallion Rice (Stir-fry classic)

Nutritional Info (per serving)
Calories: 425 kcal | Protein: 24 g | Potassium: 268 mg | Phosphorus: 255 mg | Sodium: 105 mg | Fat: 26 g | Carbs: 23 g | Cholesterol: 227 mg | Oxalates: 0.7 mg

Creativity TWIST:
Top with sliced scallions or substitute cauliflower rice. Add fresh cilantro or lime for brightness.

Parisian Herb Beef & Bell Pepper

Servings	Prep Time	Cook time	PROTEIN	PHOSPHORUS	SODIUM	POTASSIUM
2	10'	20'	MID	LOW	LOW	LOW

INGREDIENTS
- 100 g lean sirloin beef, cut in strips
- 1 medium red bell pepper (150 g), deseeded
- 4 egg whites (~132 g total)
- 3 Tbsp (42 g) unsalted butter (pantry)
- 2 Tbsp (30 ml) extra virgin olive oil (pantry)
- 1 tsp herbes de Provence (or mixed dried herbs) (pantry)

DIRECTIONS
1. Preheat oven to 200 °C (400 °F).
2. Lay out two 10-inch (25 cm) foil sheets.
3. Divide beef, bell pepper, and egg whites evenly on foil sheets.
4. Drizzle each packet with 1.5 Tbsp melted butter and 1 Tbsp olive oil.
5. Sprinkle herbs on to p.
6. Seal packets; place on baking sheet; bake 18 minutes.
7. Carefully open packets and serve directly.

Recommended Side Dish
Toasted Sourdough (To absorb the juices)

Nutritional Info (per serving)
Calories: ~411 kcal | Protein: ~22.5 g | Potassium: ~388 mg | Phosphorus: ~125 mg | Sodium: ~139 mg | Fat: ~34.5 g | Carbs: ~4.5 g | Cholesterol: ~70 mg | oxal. 4mg

Creativity TWIST:
Add 1 tsp Dijon mustard before sealing or swap red bell pepper for yellow for sweetness.

ARE YOU FINDING THIS BOOK HELPFUL? I'D LOVE TO HEAR WHAT YOU THINK.

I personally read every review, and your feedback means the world to me.It only takes 30 seconds to leave a reivew.

It truly makes a huge difference for a small author like me, and it helps other CKD warriors discover this book too.

Here's how you can leave a review for the paperback:
- **Option 1: Scan the QR code** to go straight to the review page.

- Option 2: Go to your Amazon orders, find this book, and click "Write a product review."

Option 3: Search for the book title on Amazon, scroll down to the "Customer Reviews" section, and click "Write a Review."**Once you're there, choose a star rating, a quick story about your experience, and submit!**
THAT'S IT!

Thank you so much and hope to see you in our grou p.

/ MARIANNE <3

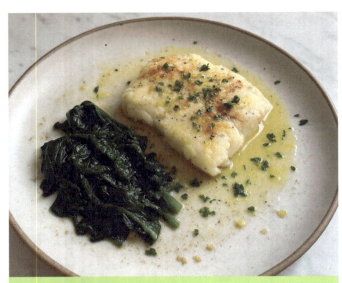

Recommended Side Dish
Roasted Cauliflower "Popcorn" (Texture contrast)

Nutritional Info (per serving)
Calories: 450 kcal | Protein: 17.3 g | Potassium: 433 mg
| Phosphorus: 200 mg | Sodium: 169 mg | Fat: 43 g |
Carbs: 2.5 g | Cholesterol: 76 mg | Oxalates: 13 mg

Creativity TWIST:
Swap parsley for fresh dill or basil; add a dusting of smoked paprika for color.

Atlantic Breeze Lemon Cod

Servings	Prep Time	Cook time	PROTEIN	PHOSPHORUS	SODIUM	POTASSIUM
2	8'	12'	MID	LOW	MID	LOW

INGREDIENTS
- 3 oz (85 g) raw cod fillet, thawed
- ½ lemon juice + zest (about 1 small lemon)
- 1 Tbsp (14 g) unsalted butter (pantry)
- 2¼ Tbsp (33 ml) olive oil (pantry)
- ½ cup (15 g) raw baby spinach, shredded
- 1 Tbsp (4 g) chopped fresh parsley
- Pinch black pepper and garlic (pantry)

DIRECTIONS
1. Warm olive oil and butter in skillet over medium heat.
2. Season cod with pepper and garlic powder.
3. Sear cod 3 minutes per side, spooning oil over fish.
4. Add spinach beside fish; squeeze lemon juice and add zest. Cover 2 minutes.
5. Remove fish and spinach; sprinkle parsley and drizzle sauce over fish.
6. Season with pepper and salt substitute to taste. Serve immediately.

Cape Ann Herb-Crusted Cod

Servings	Prep Time	Cook time	PROTEIN	PHOSPHORUS	SODIUM	POTASSIUM
1	8'	12'	MID	LOW	LOW	LOW

INGREDIENTS
- 3 oz (85 g) cod fish loin (the most tender part of the fish)
- 2 Tbsp (15 g) panko breadcrumbs (no-salt)
- 1 tsp (1 g) dried Italian herb mix
- 1 Tbsp (5 g) grated Parmesan (adds crunch)
- 1 Tbsp (15 g) mayonnaise (binds crust)
- 1 Tbsp (15 ml) extra virgin olive oil (pantry)
- Black pepper (to taste) (pantry)

DIRECTIONS
1. Preheat oven or toaster oven to 425 °F (218 °C).
2. In a small bowl, mix breadcrumbs, herbs, and Parmesan.
3. Brush cod with EVOO, then spread mayonnaise over the to p.
4. Press crumb mixture on top of the fish.
5. Place on lightly brusedh oiled foil and bake for 12–15 minutes until flaky.

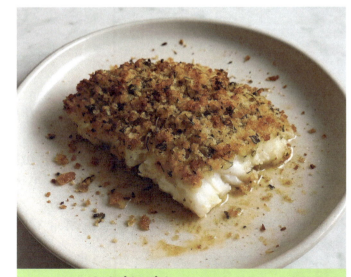

Recommended Side Dish
Blistered Green Beans (Fresh and crunchy)

Nutritional Info (per serving)
Calories: 455 kcal | Protein: 22 g | Potassium: 260 mg
| Phosphorus: 190 mg | Sodium: 180 mg | Fat: 32 g |
Carbs: 14 g | Cholesterol: 60 mg | Oxalates: <50 mg

Creativity TWIST:
Use crushed unsalted corn flakes instead of panko for a different crunch.

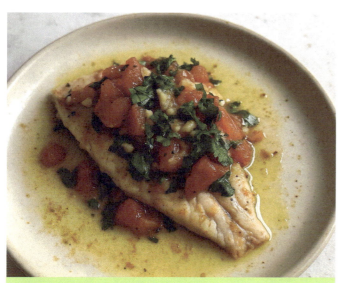

Recommended Side Dish
Lemon-Parsley White Rice (Light and citrusy)

Nutritional Info (per serving)
Calories: 445 kcal | Protein: 17.3 g | Potassium: 363 mg |
Phosphorus: 190 mg | Sodium: 50 mg | Fat: 43 g | Carbs:
2.6 g | Cholesterol: 34 mg | Oxalates: ~9.5 mg

Gulf Coast Garlic Snapper Packets

Servings	Prep Time	Cook time	PROTEIN	PHOSPHORUS	SODIUM	POTASSIUM
1	5'	15'	MID	LOW	LOW	MID

INGREDIENTS
- 2.5 oz (71 g) red snapper fillet, raw
- 3 Tbsp (45 g) diced ripe, peeled tomatoes
- 1 Tbsp (4 g) chopped cilantro
- 1 tsp (3 g) minced garlic
- 3 Tbsp (42 ml) olive oil (main fat component) (pantry)
- Pinch black pepper (pantry)

DIRECTIONS
1. On a sheet of foil, drizzle olive oil, then place fish on foil.
2. Top fish with tomatoes, garlic, and cilantro.
3. Cover and seal the foil packet tightly.
4. Bake at 400 °F (200 °C) for 15 minutes or grill.
5. Remove from oven, carefully open packet, and serve.

Creativity TWIST:
Add a few capers (watch sodium) for briny pop and/or a squeeze of lime. Or ⅓ cup black olives.

Bay-Island Coconut Catfish Skillet

Servings	Prep Time	Cook time	PROTEIN	PHOSPHORUS	SODIUM	POTASSIUM
1	7'	12'	MID	LOW	LOW	MID

INGREDIENTS
- 3 oz (85 g) catfish strips, uncooked
- ¼ cup (60 ml) lite canned coconut milk
- 1 Tbsp (15 ml) minced red bell pepper, peeled
- 1 tsp (5 ml) grated fresh ginger
- 3 Tbsp (45 ml) olive oil (1 tsp for sauté + 2 Tbsp added for calories) (pantry)
- 1 Tbsp (4 g) chopped green onion tops

DIRECTIONS
1. Pour ¼ cup boiling water over grated ginger; let sit 3–5 minutes.
2. Strain ginger water. Sauté ginger in 1 tsp olive oil, 30 seconds high heat.
3. Add catfish and ginger water; cook 3 minutes medium heat.
4. Pour coconut milk; simmer 6 minutes.
5. Add bell pepper and green onion; cook 2mins.
6. Drizzle 2 tbsp olive oil before serving.

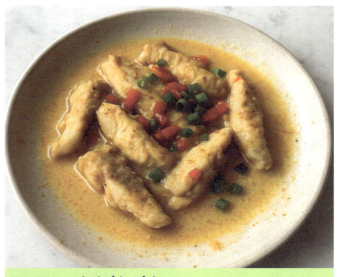

Recommended Side Dish
Sautéed Cabbage w/ Vinegar (Acid cuts the fat)

Nutritional Info (per serving)
Calories: 437 kcal | Protein: 21 g | Potassium: 432 mg |
Phosphorus: 212 mg | Sodium: 73 mg | Fat: 39 g | Carbs:
3 g | Cholesterol: 60 mg | Oxalates: <50 mg

Creativity TWIST:
Replace catfish with swai or tilapia. Garnish with toasted unsweetened coconut flakes.

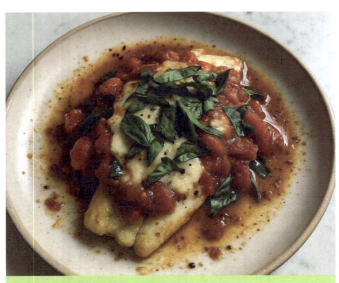

Recommended Side Dish
Herbed Golden Couscous (Mediterranean style)

Nutritional Info (per serving)
Calories: 462 kcal | Protein: 20.4 g | Potassium: 375 mg
| Phosphorus: 252 mg | Sodium: 164 mg | Fat: 20.4 g |
Carbs: 3.7 g | Cholesterol: 55 mg | Oxalates: <5 mg

Monterey Bay Tomato-Basil Flounder

Servings	Prep Time	Cook time	PROTEIN	PHOSPHORUS	SODIUM	POTASSIUM
1	10'	15'	MID	LOW	LOW	LOW

INGREDIENTS
- 3 oz (85 g) flounder fillet, uncooked
- ¼ cup (60 g) no-salt diced tomatoes, drained
- 1 Tbsp (4 g) fresh basil, cut in ribbons
- 1 tsp (5 ml) balsamic vinegar
- 1 Tbsp (8 g) shredded part-skim mozzarella cheese
- 3 Tbsp (45 ml) olive oil (pantry)
- Fresh ground pepper, to taste (pantry)

DIRECTIONS
1. Heat small skillet over medium-high heat for 1 minute.
2. Sear fillet 2 minutes per side in olive oil.
3. Add tomatoes and vinegar to skillet over fish. Cover pan and cook 4 minutes on medium heat.
4. Add mozzarella and basil ribbons. Cover and let cheese melt for 2 minutes.

Creativity TWIST:
Use oregano instead of basil for pizza-style flavor. Try a splash of lemon juice for citrus zing.

Chesapeake Garden Tuna Patties

Servings	Prep Time	Cook time	PROTEIN	PHOSPHORUS	SODIUM	POTASSIUM
2	8'	12'	MID	LOW	LOW	LOW

INGREDIENTS
- 6 oz (170 g) canned light tuna in water, no-salt, drained
- 1 Tbsp (9 g) finely minced celery hearts
- 2 Tbsp (12 g) no-salt breadcrumbs
- 1.5 large egg whites (approx. 50 g)
- 4 Tbsp (54 ml) olive oil (pantry)
- Old Bay-style seasoning (pantry)
- Black pepper (pantry)
- Olive oil spray (pantry)

DIRECTIONS
1. Mix all ingredients in a medium bowl.
2. Form two patties.
3. Pan-sear in lightly oiled skillet, cooking 4 minutes per side.
4. Serve immediately.

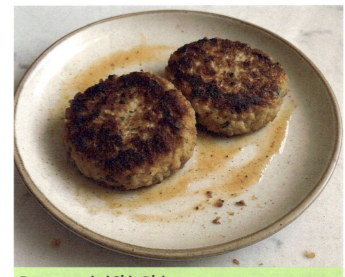

Recommended Side Dish
Cucumber & Onion Vinegar Salad (Fresh pickle vibe)

Nutritional Info (per serving)
Calories: 451 kcal | Protein: 21.7 g | Potassium: 180 mg
| Phosphorus: 133 mg | Sodium: 115 mg | Fat: 24.5 g |
Carbs: 4.25 g | Cholesterol: 13 mg | Oxalates: 0.5 mg

Creativity TWIST:
Serve on small toasted slider bun with lettuce for handheld meal.

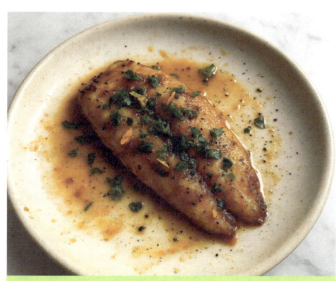

Recommended Side Dish
Asian-Style Sesame-Scallion Rice (Ginger match)

Nutritional Info (per serving)
Calories: 460 kcal | Protein: 18.7 g | Potassium: 325 mg | Phosphorus: 190 mg | Sodium: 59 mg | Fat: 28 g | Carbs: 12.5 g | Cholesterol: 55 mg | Oxalates: 10 mg

Citrus-Ginger Swai Fillet

Servings	Prep Time	Cook time	PROTEIN	PHOSPHORUS	SODIUM	POTASSIUM
1	5'	15'	MID	LOW	LOW	LOW

INGREDIENTS
- 3 oz (85 g) swai (pangasius) fillet, uncooked
- 1 Tbsp (15 ml) fresh lemon juice
- ½ tsp grated orange zest
- 1 tsp fresh grated ginger
- 2 tsp honey (pantry)
- 1 Tbsp (1 g) chopped cilantro
- 2 Tbsp (30 ml) olive oil (pantry)

DIRECTIONS
1. Heat 2 Tbsp olive oil in small skillet over medium-high heat.
2. Sear swai fillet 3 minutes per side until cooked and browned.
3. In small bowl, whisk lemon juice, honey, and grated ginger.
4. Pour glaze over fish in skillet. Simmer 5 minutes until thickened.
5. Remove from heat, top with orange zest and chopped cilantro. Season with pepper.

Creativity TWIST:
Add pinch crushed red pepper for heat. Serve with 2 large strawberries or cucumber slices.

Cajun Red Drum Sauté

Servings	Prep Time	Cook time	PROTEIN	PHOSPHORUS	SODIUM	POTASSIUM
1	7'	10'	MID	LOW	LOW	MID

INGREDIENTS
- 2.5 oz (71 g) red drum (or redfish) fillet, uncooked
- 1 tsp Cajun spice (salt-free) (pantry)
- 2 Tbsp (15 g) sliced zucchini, peeled
- 2 Tbsp (30 g) diced onion
- 3 Tbsp (42 g) unsalted butter (pantry)
- 1 tsp (5 ml) olive oil (pantry)

DIRECTIONS
1. Place fish on plate; dust with Cajun spice.
2. In small skillet, melt butter and olive oil. Cook onions over medium-high heat 2 minutes.
3. Add zucchini; cook 3 minutes more.
4. Push vegetables aside, add fish; cook 3 minutes.
5. Flip fish; cook 3 minutes more.
6. Sear fish over vegetables before serving.

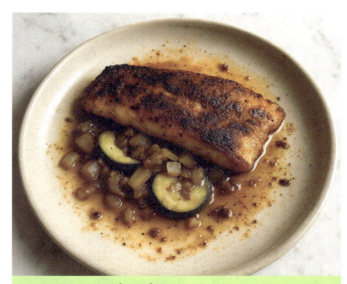

Recommended Side Dish
Zucchini & Corn Sauté (Cajun classic veggies)

Nutritional Info (per serving)
Calories: 442 kcal | Protein: 18 g | Potassium: 411 mg | Phosphorus: 196 mg | Sodium: 57 mg | Fat: 41 g | Carbs: 4 g | Cholesterol: 107 mg | Oxalates: 14 mg

Creativity TWIST:
Add lemon juice for brightness or thyme for Creole flair. Swap zucchini for yellow squash or parsley.

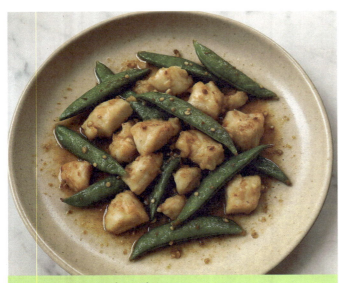

Recommended Side Dish
Roasted Cauliflower "Popcorn" (Adds crunch)

Nutritional Info (per serving)
Calories: 504 kcal | Protein: 22 g | Potassium: 460 mg
| Phosphorus: 196 mg | Sodium: 198 mg | Fat: 40.6 g |
Carbs: 6.5 g | Cholesterol: 50 mg | Oxalates: 3 mg

Creativity TWIST:
Sprinkle with sesame seeds (pantry) or substitute orange juice for lime for sweetness.

Sesame-Lime Pollock Stir-Fry

Servings	Prep Time	Cook time	PROTEIN	PHOSPHORUS	SODIUM	POTASSIUM
1	8'	10'	MID	LOW	LOW	LOW

INGREDIENTS
- 3 oz (85 g) Alaskan pollock chunks, uncooked
- 2/3 cup (65 g) sugar-snap pea pods, cut lengthwise
- 1 tsp (5 ml) low-sodium soy sauce
- 1 tsp (4.5 ml) toasted sesame oil (pantry)
- 2.5 Tbsp (37.5 ml) olive oil (pantry)
- Juice of ½ lime (~15 g)

DIRECTIONS
1. Heat sesame oil and olive oil in skillet with sugar-snap peas for 2 minutes.
2. Add pollock; cook 3 minutes per side.
3. Add soy sauce and lime juice; cook 3 more minutes.

Mustard-Maple Rainbow Trout

Servings	Prep Time	Cook time	PROTEIN	PHOSPHORUS	SODIUM	POTASSIUM
1	8'	12'	MID	LOW	LOW	LOW

INGREDIENTS
- 85 g (3 oz) rainbow trout fillet (skin removed for easier chewing)
- 1 Tbsp (20 g) pure maple syrup
- 1 tsp (5 g) Dijon mustard
- 1 Tbsp (15 ml) olive oil
- 1 tsp (5 ml) apple cider vinegar

DIRECTIONS
1. Pat trout dry, season with black pepper.
2. Whisk maple syrup, Dijon mustard, and apple cider vinegar.
3. Heat olive oil in a non-stick skillet over medium.
4. Cook trout 4 minutes until golden and flaky, then fli p.
5. Lower heat, brush mustard-maple sauce on top, cook 3-4 more minutes until done.
6. Remove from heat and drizzle remaining sauce over trout before serving.serving.

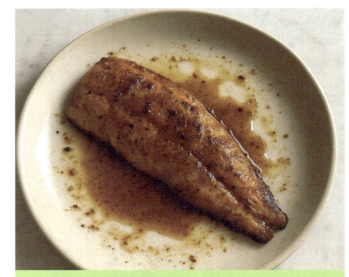

Recommended Side Dish
Blistered Green Beans (Classic fish side)

Nutritional Info (per serving)
Calories: 470 kcal | Protein: 20 g | Potassium: 320 mg
| Phosphorus: 214 mg | Sodium: 108 mg | Fat: 38 g |
Carbs: 14 g | Cholesterol: 55 mg | Oxalates: 0 mg

Creativity TWIST:
Swap apple cider vinegar with lemon juice. Or serve alongside soft mashed cauliflower.

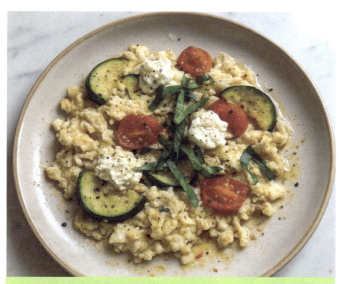

Recommended Side Dish
Toasted Sourdough (Great for dipping)

Nutritional Info (per serving)
Calories: 491 kcal | Protein: 22 g | Potassium: 562 mg | Phosphorus: 182 mg | Sodium: 279 mg | Fat: 42 g | Carbs: 6 g | Cholesterol: 32 mg | Oxalates: 11 mg

Verona Egg-White Ricotta Zucchini

Servings	Prep Time	Cook time	PROTEIN	PHOSPHORUS	SODIUM	POTASSIUM
1	8'	10'	LOW	LOW	LOW	LOW

INGREDIENTS
- 4 large pasteurized egg whites (about ½ cup) (132 g)
- ¼ medium zucchini, sliced thin (½ cup) (60 g)
- ¼ cup part-skim, unsalted ricotta cheese (62 g)
- ¼ cup quartered cherry tomatoes (37 g)
- 2½ Tbsp olive oil (EVOO preferred) (37 ml) (Pantry)
- 2 Tbsp fresh basil ribbons (8 g)

DIRECTIONS
1. Heat 2½ Tbsp olive oil in a medium non-stick skillet.
2. Sauté zucchini for 2 minutes. Add tomatoes, cook 1 minute.
3. Pour in egg whites, stir and cook over medium heat until softly set, about 4–5 minutes.
4. Fold in ricotta, cook 30 seconds more.
5. Top with basil ribbons and black pepper

Creativity TWIST:
Replace basil with fresh mint. Drizzle ½ tsp (1.7 ml) honey for a "sweet-savory" Tuscan vibe

Santa Fe Egg-White & Tofu Pepper Toss

Servings	Prep Time	Cook time	PROTEIN	PHOSPHORUS	SODIUM	POTASSIUM
1	5'	12'	LOW	LOW	LOW	MID

INGREDIENTS
- 4 large egg whites (132g)
- 0.5 oz firm tofu, cut into tiny cubes (14g)
- ¼ cup cauliflower rice (28.5g)
- 2 Tbsp diced red bell pepper (18g)
- 2 Tbsp chopped cilantro (2g)
- 3 Tbsp olive oil (40.5 ml)

DIRECTIONS
1. Heat 3 Tbsp olive oil in small pan; sauté pepper & cauliflower 3 min.
2. Add tofu. Cook 2 min.
3. Stir in egg whites; scramble until set.
4. Sprinkle cilantro and a dash of cumin

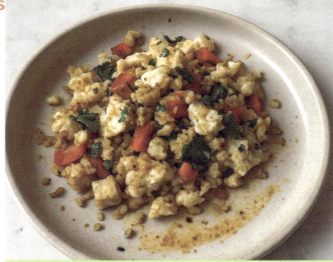

Recommended Side Dish
Lemon-Parsley White Rice (Makes it a bowl)

Nutritional Info (per cakelet)
Calories: 463 kcal | Protein: 17.7 g | Potassium: 452 mg | Phosphorus: 107 mg | Sodium: 235 mg | Fat: 42 g | Carbs: 5.1 g | Cholesterol: 0 mg | Oxalates: ~3 mg

Creativity TWIST:
Serve over crisp butter lettuce with a lime juice for fajita flair or add a pinch of smoked paprika

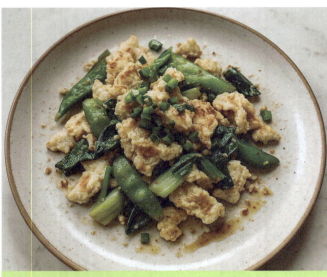

Recommended Side Dish
Asian-Style Sesame-Scallion Rice

Nutritional Info (per serving)
Calories: ~475 kcal | Protein: 16.4 g | Potassium: 418 mg | Phosphorus: 110 mg | Sodium: 230 mg | Fat: 33.5 g | Carbs: 6 g | Cholesterol: 0 mg | Oxalates: ~14 mg

Creativity TWIST:
Sprinkle toasted sesame seeds or grate a whisper of yuzu zest for brightness.

Kyoto Ginger Egg Mushroom Stir-Fry

Servings	Prep Time	Cook time	PROTEIN	PHOSPHORUS	SODIUM	POTASSIUM
1	7'	10'	MID	LOW	LOW	MID

INGREDIENTS
- 4 large egg whites (132 g)
- ½ cup bok choy, chopped (43 g) - (Or mushrooms to lower potassium even more)
- 2 Tbsp snow-pea halves (20 g)
- 1 Tbsp freshly minced ginger (6 g)
- 3 Tbsp unsalted butter (45 ml) (Pantry)
- 2 Tbsp sliced green onion (12 g)

DIRECTIONS
1. Warm 3 Tbsp unsalted butter in a pan over medium heat. Stir-fry minced ginger for 30 seconds.
2. Add bok choy and snow peas; cook 3-4 minutes until tender.
3. Pour in egg whites and gently stir until fluffy and cooked through.
4. Top with sliced green onions and a dash of low-sodium soy sauce if desired.

Guten Garden Egg-White Frittata

Servings	Prep Time	Cook time	PROTEIN	PHOSPHORUS	SODIUM	POTASSIUM
1	8'	12'	MID	LOW	LOW	MID

INGREDIENTS
- 4 large egg whites (132 g)
- 1 large whole egg (50 g)
- 2.5 Tbsp diced baby bella mushrooms (10 g)
- 2 Tbsp diced red bell pepper (18 g)
- 0.3 oz low-sodium goat cheese (9 g)
- 2 Tbsp olive oil (27 ml) (Pantry)
- 2 Tbsp chopped fresh parsley (8 g)

DIRECTIONS
1. Heat 2 Tbsp olive oil in an 8-inch oven-safe pan over medium heat.
2. Cook mushrooms and red bell pepper for 3 minutes until softened.
3. Pour in egg whites and whole egg; stir gently to combine.
4. Add goat cheese on to p.
5. Broil for 5-6 minutes until firm.
6. Garnish with chopped fresh parsley

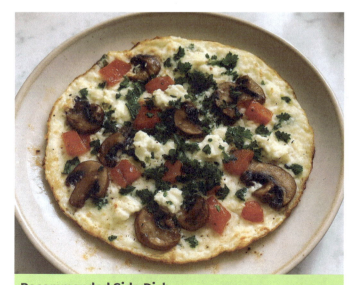

Recommended Side Dish
Roasted Red Pepper & Onion (Flavor boost)

Nutritional Info (per serving)
Calories: 485 kcal | Protein: 20.3 g | Potassium: 470 mg | Phosphorus: 230 mg | Sodium: 390 mg | Fat: 31 g | Carbs: 4.5 g | Cholesterol: 190 mg | Oxalates: 10 mg

Creativity TWIST:
Add smoked paprika or thyme for rustic notes. Swap goat cheese for soft ricotta for creaminess.

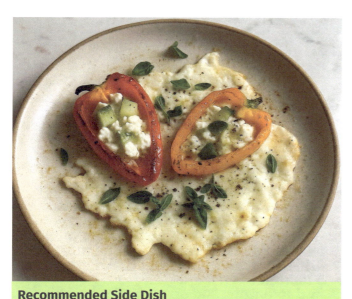

Recommended Side Dish
Garlic-Infused Penne (Makes it a full meal)

Nutritional Info (per serving)

Calories: 454 kcal | Protein: 17.5 g | Potassium: 406 mg | Phosphorus: 107 mg | Sodium: 263 mg | Fat: 40 g | Carbs: 8.6 g | Cholesterol: 4 mg | Oxalates: 2 mg

Catalina Cottage-Stuffed Mini Peppers

Servings	Prep Time	Cook time	PROTEIN	PHOSPHORUS	SODIUM	POTASSIUM
1	10'	12'	MID	LOW	LOW	LOW

INGREDIENTS
- 3 large egg whites (about 99 g)
- 2 mini sweet peppers, deseeded and halved (60 g)
- 3 Tbsp low-sodium cottage cheese (45 g)
- ¼ cup diced cucumber (30 g)
- 1.5 Tbsp olive oil (22 ml) (Pantry)
- 1 Tbsp unsalted butter (15 ml) (Pantry)
- 1 Tbsp fresh oregano leaves (3 g)

DIRECTIONS
1. Sear mini peppers cut-side down in 1.5 Tbsp olive oil for 3 minutes; flip and cook briefly.
2. Spoon cottage cheese and diced cucumber into pepper cavities.
3. Pour egg whites around peppers, cover, and cook 5-6 minutes until egg whites set.
4. Add unsalted butter and let it melt over the dish.
5. Sprinkle fresh oregano leaves and cracked black pepper to taste.

Creativity TWIST:
Dust with za'atar and drizzle ½ tsp (1.7 ml) honey for a Mediterranean sweet kick.

Boulder BBQ Seitan & Pepper Skillet

Servings	Prep Time	Cook time	PROTEIN	PHOSPHORUS	SODIUM	POTASSIUM
2	7'	10'	MID	LOW	LOW	LOW

INGREDIENTS
- 2¼ oz (64 g) plain seitan strips
- ½ cup (35 g) iceberg lettuce, chopped
- ½ cup (90 g) yellow squash, diced
- 2 Tbsp (30 g) no-salt tomato purée
- 1 Tbsp (6 g) chopped green onion
- 2½ Tbsp extra virgin olive oil (37 ml) (Pantry)

DIRECTIONS
1. Warm 2½ Tbsp olive oil in a skillet on medium heat.
2. Sear seitan strips for 2 minutes. Add iceberg lettuce and yellow squash; cook for 3 minutes.
3. Stir in tomato purée. Simmer for 2 minutes to glaze.
4. Finish with green onion and cracked pepper.

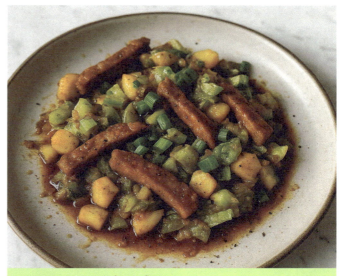

Recommended Side Dish
Sautéed Cabbage w/ Vinegar (Like BBQ & Slaw)

Nutritional Info (per serving)

Calories: 480 kcal | Protein: 16 g | Potassium: 283 mg | Phosphorus: 85 mg | Sodium: 50 mg | Fat: 37 g | Carbs: 10 g | Cholesterol: 0 mg | Oxalates: 16 mg

Creativity TWIST:
Splash ½ tsp apple-cider vinegar plus a pinch of smoked paprika for backyard BBQ taste.

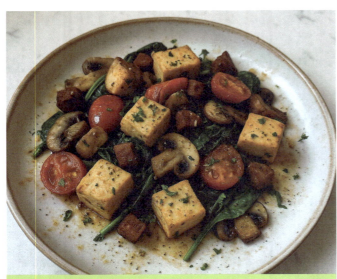

Recommended Side Dish
Leached Garlic Mashed Potatoes (Hearty dinner)

Nutritional Info (per serving)
Calories: ~366 kcal | Protein: 19.5 g | Potassium: 560 mg | Phosphorus: 205 mg | Sodium: 325 mg | Fat: 30 g | Carbs: 7 g | Cholesterol: 0 mg | Oxalates: ~49 mg

Creativity TWIST:
Replace parsley with dill. Drizzle ½ tsp honey mustard for a wine country vibe.

Big Bear Herb Tofu-Seitan Sauté

Servings	Prep Time	Cook time	PROTEIN	PHOSPHORUS	SODIUM	POTASSIUM
1	6'	9'	MID	MID	MID	MID

INGREDIENTS
- 3 oz (85 g) seitan, diced
- ½ cup (36 g) sliced cremini mushrooms
- ¼ cup (7.5 g) baby spinach, raw
- ¼ cup (37 g) halved grape tomatoes
- 2 Tbsp (28 g) olive oil (pantry)
- Chopped fresh parsley
- Optional: ¼ cup (43 g) cooked quinoa

DIRECTIONS
1. Heat olive oil in medium pan over medium heat. Sauté mushrooms for 2 minutes.
2. Add seitan and cook until browned, about 5 minutes.
3. Add tomatoes and spinach. Cook until spinach wilts, about 2 minutes.
4. Optionally stir in cooked quinoa for extra calories and texture.
5. Season with parsley, lemon and black pepper.

Valletta White-Bean & Seitan Stew

Servings	Prep Time	Cook time	PROTEIN	PHOSPHORUS	SODIUM	POTASSIUM
1	8'	12'	MID	LOW	LOW	MID

INGREDIENTS
- 1.2 oz seitan, diced (34 g)
- ¼ cup no-salt cannellini beans, rinsed (43 g)
- ¼ cup no-salt diced tomatoes (61 g)
- ¼ cup diced zucchini (45 g)
- 1 Tbsp finely chopped red onion (15 g)
- 2½ Tbsp olive oil (37.5 ml) (Pantry)
- Splash of red-wine vinegar (Pantry)
- Dried oregano (Pantry)

DIRECTIONS
1. Heat 2 tbsp EVOO in a saucepan.
2. Sauté red onion and seitan for 2 minutes.
3. Add zucchini; cook 2 minutes on medium heat.
4. Stir in cannellini beans, diced tomatoes, and ¼ cup water; simmer 6 minutes until thickened.
5. Drizzle with remaining ½ tbsp EVOO.
6. Top with oregano and a splash of red-wine vinegar.

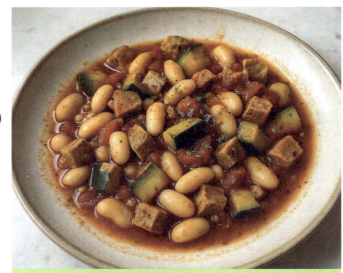

Recommended Side Dish
Toasted Sourdough (Stew needs bread)

Nutritional Info (per serving)
Calories: 468 kcal | Protein: 18.5 g | Potassium: 560 mg | Phosphorus: 140 mg | Sodium: 15 mg | Fat: 36.7 g | Carbs: 21 g | Cholesterol: 0 mg | Oxalates: 9 mg

Creativity TWIST:
Ladle stew over ¼ cup cooked couscous for a Maltese market feel.basil for a different aroma.

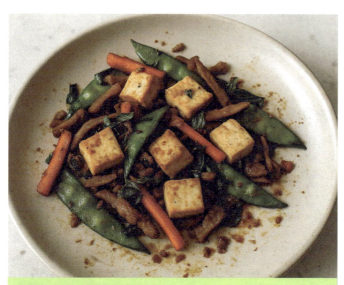

Recommended Side Dish
Asian-Style Sesame-Scallion Rice

Nutritional Info (per serving)
Calories: 436 kcal | Protein: 21.4 g | Potassium: 332 mg
| Phosphorus: 174 mg | Sodium: 199 mg | Fat: 36 g |
Carbs: 14.6 g | Cholesterol: 0 mg | Oxalates: ~18 mg

Bangkok Basil Tofu-Seitan Stir-Fry

Servings	Prep Time	Cook time	PROTEIN	PHOSPHORUS	SODIUM	POTASSIUM
1	7'	8'	MID	LOW	LOW	LOW

INGREDIENTS
- 4 oz extra-firm tofu, cubed (113 g)
- 0.5 oz seitan, slivered (14 g)
- ½ cup snow pea halves (50 g)
- ¼ cup carrot sticks (30 g)
- 2 Tbsp chopped Thai basil (5 g)
- 2 Tbsp olive oil (27 ml) (Pantry)
- 1 tsp rice vinegar (5 ml) (Pantry)

DIRECTIONS
1. Add 1 Tbsp olive oil, snow peas, and carrots to a wok; cook for 1 minute.
2. Add tofu, seitan, chopped basil, and ginger; stir-fry for 4 minutes until lightly browned.
3. Splash in 1 tsp rice vinegar and stir.
4. Drizzle remaining 1 Tbsp olive oil over before serving or use it for cooking if preferred.

Creativity TWIST:
Top with 1 tsp crushed unsalted cashews and a squeeze of lime for street food flair.

Napa Chickpea-Zucchini Cakes

Servings	Prep Time	Cook time	PROTEIN	PHOSPHORUS	SODIUM	POTASSIUM
1	10'	10'	MID	LOW	LOW	MID

INGREDIENTS
- ¾ cup no-salt chickpeas, rinsed and mashed (about 122 g)
- 1 oz seitan, minced (28 g)
- 3 Tbsp grated zucchini, squeezed dry (~22 g)
- 1 Tbsp finely diced red bell pepper (~9 g)
- 1 Tbsp chopped parsley (~3.8 g)
- 1½ Tbsp olive oil (20 ml) (Pantry)
- Dash of lemon juice (Pantry)

DIRECTIONS
1. Combine chickpeas, seitan, grated zucchini, and diced red bell pepper in a bowl.
2. Mix well and form two 3-inch patties. Chill for 3 minutes.
3. Pan-sear patties in skillet with 1½ Tbsp olive oil, cooking 3 minutes per side until golden brown.
4. Sprinkle chopped parsley and a dash of lemon juice before serving.

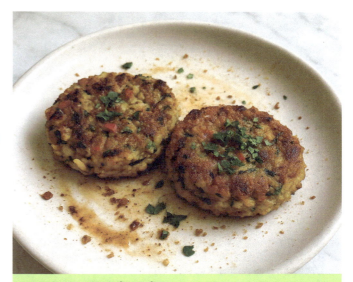

Recommended Side Dish
Cucumber & Onion Vinegar Salad (Bright finish)

Nutritional Info (per serving)
Calories: 484 kcal | Protein: 20 g | Potassium: 378 mg
| Phosphorus: 157 mg | Sodium: 145 mg | Fat: 23 g |
Carbs: 34 g | Cholesterol: 0 mg | Oxalates: ~40 mg

Creativity TWIST:
Serve with a dollop of low-sugar peach salsa for a sunny California note or fresh mint for brightness.

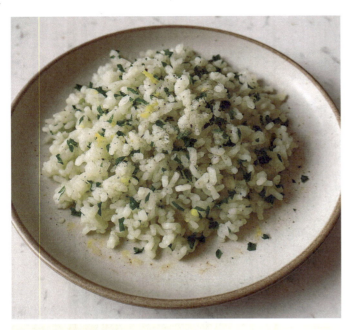

Lemon-Parsley White Rice

Servings	Prep Time	Cook time	PROTEIN	PHOSPHORUS	SODIUM	K POTASSIUM
2	5'	20'	LOW	LOW	LOW	LOW

INGREDIENTS
- ½ cup White rice (long grain or jasmine, dry)
- 1 cup Water
- 1.5 tbsp Unsalted butter (or olive oil)
- ½ Lemon (zested and juiced)
- ¼ cup Fresh parsley (chopped fine)
- ¼ tsp Black pepper

DIRECTIONS
1. Rinse the rice thoroughly in cold water until the water runs clear.
2. In a small pot, bring water to a boil. Add rice, reduce heat to low, cover tightly, and simmer for 18–20 minutes.
3. Remove from heat and let sit, covered, for 5 minutes.
4. Fluff with a fork. Stir in the butter, lemon juice, lemon zest, and black pepper.
5. Gently fold in the fresh parsley right before serving.

Nutritional Info (per serving)
Calories: 235kcal | Protein: 3.5g | Potassium: 60mg | Phosphorus: 55mg | Sodium: 5mg | Fat: 9g | Carbs: 38g | Cholesterol: 22mg | Oxalates: Low

Creativity TWIST:
Add a pinch of saffron threads to the boiling water for a vibrant yellow color and earthy flavor.

Garlic-Infused Penne Pasta

Servings	Prep Time	Cook time	PROTEIN	PHOSPHORUS	SODIUM	K POTASSIUM
2	5'	12'	LOW	LOW	LOW	LOW

INGREDIENTS
- 4 oz White Penne or Bowtie pasta (dry)
- 1.5 tbsp Olive oil
- 2 cloves Garlic (crushed or thinly sliced)
- ¼ tsp Red pepper flakes
- 1 tbsp Fresh basil (chopped)

DIRECTIONS
1. Bring a pot of water to a boil. Add pasta and cook according to package directions. Do not salt the water.
2. While pasta cooks, combine olive oil and garlic in a small skillet over very low heat. Sizzle gently for 5 minutes to infuse.
3. Drain pasta well.
4. Toss hot pasta immediately with garlic oil and red pepper flakes.
5. Top with fresh basil.

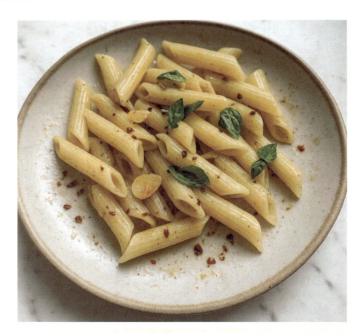

Nutritional Info (per serving)
Calories: 290kcal | Protein: 7g | Potassium: 60mg | Phosphorus: 100mg | Sodium: 2mg | Fat: 10g | Carbs: 42g | Cholesterol: 0mg | Oxalates: Low

Creativity TWIST:
Toss with 1 tablespoon of toasted pine nuts for texture.

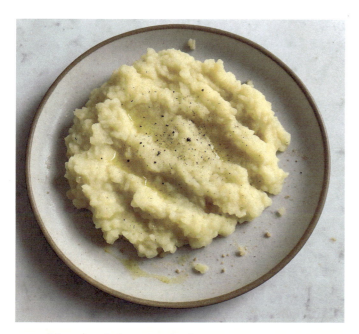

Leached "Creamy" Garlic Mashed

Servings	Prep Time	Cook time	PROTEIN	PHOSPHORUS	SODIUM	K POTASSIUM
2	4h	20'	LOW	LOW	LOW	MID

INGREDIENTS
- 1 large Russet potato (approx 300g, peeled and diced into 1-inch cubes)
- 4 cups Warm water (for soaking)
- 1.5 tbsp Unsalted butter
- 2 tbsp Rice milk (or non-dairy creamer)
- ½ tsp Garlic powder (optional pantry)
- ¼ tsp Onion powder (optional pantry)
- Black pepper (optional pantry)

DIRECTIONS
1. Leaching: Peel and dice potato. Soak in warm water for at least 4 hours to reduce potassium.
2. Drain and rinse potato cubes.
3. Boil in fresh water for 15 minutes until very tender. Drain well.
4. Mash thoroughly.
5. Stir in butter, rice milk, garlic powder, onion powder, and pepper until smooth.

Nutritional Info (per serving)
Calories: 205kcal | Protein: 3g | Potassium: 320mg | Phosphorus: 75mg | Sodium: 10mg | Fat: 9g | Carbs: 28g | Cholesterol: 22mg | Oxalates: Moderate

Creativity TWIST:
Add 1 tablespoon of snipped fresh chives for an oniony bite that looks beautiful against the mash

Toasted Sourdough Garlic "Points"

Servings	Prep Time	Cook time	PROTEIN	PHOSPHORUS	SODIUM	K POTASSIUM
2	5'	5'	LOW	LOW	MID	LOW

INGREDIENTS
- 2 large slices Sourdough bread (thick slices)
- 1.5 tbsp Olive oil
- 1 clove Raw garlic (peeled)
- ½ tsp Dried oregano
- Paprika

DIRECTIONS
1. Preheat broiler. Slice bread diagonally into triangles.
2. Brush both sides generously with olive oil.
3. Broil for 2–3 minutes until golden brown (watch closely).
4. While hot, rub the raw garlic clove vigorously over the rough bread surface.
5. Sprinkle with oregano and paprika.

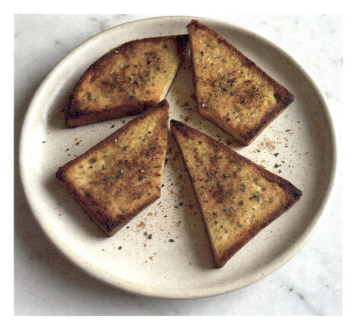

Nutritional Info (per serving)
Calories: 200kcal | Protein: 4g | Potassium: 65mg | Phosphorus: 50mg | Sodium: 200mg | Fat: 10g | Carbs: 28g | Cholesterol: 0mg | Oxalates: Low

Creativity TWIST:
Rub with a cut tomato slice after the garlic for a "Pan con Tomate" style moisture.

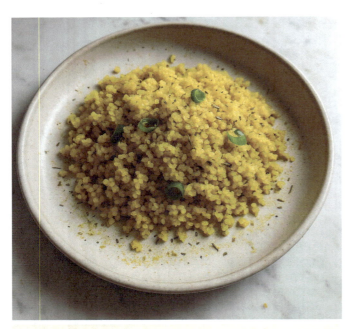

Herbed Golden Couscous

Servings	Prep Time	Cook time	PROTEIN	PHOSPHORUS	SODIUM	K POTASSIUM
2	2'	5'	LOW	LOW	LOW	LOW

INGREDIENTS
- ½ cup Couscous (dry, plain)
- ¾ cup Low-sodium vegetable broth (or water)
- 1 tbsp Olive oil (Pantry)
- ¼ tsp Turmeric powder (optional pantry)
- ½ tsp Dried thyme (optional pantry)
- 1 Green onion (sliced, green parts only)

DIRECTIONS
1. Bring broth, olive oil, turmeric, and thyme to a boil in a small saucepan.
2. Remove from heat. Stir in couscous.
3. Cover tightly and let sit for 5 minutes.
4. Fluff with a fork and stir in green onions.

Nutritional Info (per serving)
Calories: 520 kcal | Protein: 18 g | Potassium: 345 mg | Phosphorus: 220 mg | Sodium: 370 mg | Fat: 18 g | Carbs: 48 g | Cholesterol: 10 mg | Oxalates: ~8 mg

Creativity TWIST:
Try adding fresh herbs like basil or oregano for flavor without sodium.

Asian-Style Sesame-Scallion Rice

Servings	Prep Time	Cook time	PROTEIN	PHOSPHORUS	SODIUM	K POTASSIUM
1	5'	20'	LOW	LOW	LOW	LOW

INGREDIENTS
- ½ cup White rice (dry)
- 1 cup Water
- 1 tbsp Toasted sesame oil
- 1 stalk Green onion (chopped)
- ¼ tsp Ground ginger
- 1 tsp Rice vinegar

DIRECTIONS
1. Rinse rice. Boil water and rice, reduce heat, cover, and simmer 18–20 minutes.
2. Remove from heat. Drizzle with sesame oil and rice vinegar.
3. Sprinkle with ginger and fluff.
4. Fold in green onions.

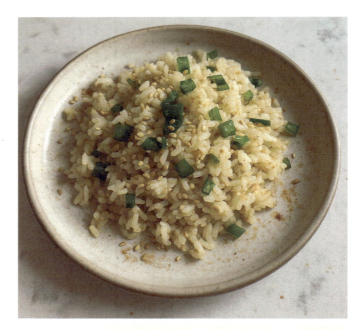

Nutritional Info (per serving)
Calories: 220kcal | Protein: 3.5g | Potassium: 55mg | Phosphorus: 55mg | Sodium: 2mg | Fat: 7g | Carbs: 38g | Cholesterol: 0mg | Oxalates: Low

Creativity TWIST:
Add chopped canned water chestnuts (drained) for a renal-safe crunch that mimics peanuts.

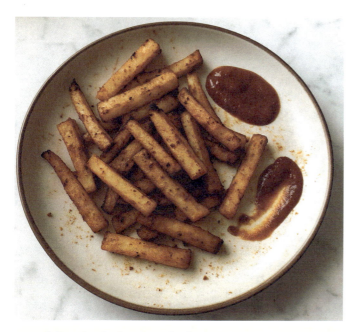

Roasted Turnip "Fries"

Servings	Prep Time	Cook time	PROTEIN	PHOSPHORUS	SODIUM	POTASSIUM
2	10'	25'	LOW	LOW	LOW	LOW

INGREDIENTS
- 2 medium Turnips (peeled, approx 300g total)
- 2.5 tbsp Vegetable oil (needed to reach calorie goal)
- ½ tsp Smoked paprika
- ¼ tsp Garlic powder
- ¼ tsp Black pepper

DIRECTIONS
1. Preheat oven to 425°F (220°C).
2. Cut peeled turnips into ½-inch sticks.
3. Toss thoroughly with oil, paprika, garlic powder, and pepper.
4. Roast on a baking sheet for 20–25 minutes, flipping halfway, until crisp-tender.

Nutritional Info (per serving)
Calories: 200kcal | Protein: 1.5g | Potassium: 285mg | Phosphorus: 40mg | Sodium: 90mg | Fat: 17g | Carbs: 9g | Cholesterol: 0mg | Oxalates: Low

Creativity TWIST:
Sprinkle with onion powder and serve with a side of malt vinegar for a "chip shop" flavor.

Roasted Cauliflower "Popcorn"

Servings	Prep Time	Cook time	PROTEIN	PHOSPHORUS	SODIUM	POTASSIUM
1	10'	25'	LOW	LOW	LOW	MID

INGREDIENTS
- ½ head Cauliflower (approx 200g usable florets)
- 2.5 tbsp Olive oil (generous coating needed for calories/crispness)
- ½ tsp Turmeric powder
- ¼ tsp Onion powder
- Black pepper

DIRECTIONS
1. Preheat oven to 400°F (200°C).
2. Cut cauliflower into small, bite-sized florets.
3. Toss with olive oil, turmeric, onion powder, and pepper.
4. Roast for 20–25 minutes until browned and crispy.

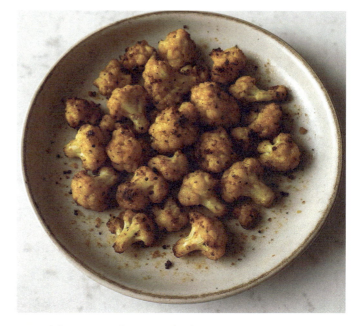

Nutritional Info (per serving)
Calories: 175kcal | Protein: 2g | Potassium: 300mg | Phosphorus: 45mg | Sodium: 30mg | Fat: 17g | Carbs: 5g | Cholesterol: 0mg | Oxalates: Low

Creativity TWIST:
Toss with a splash of Frank's RedHot (low sodium version) after roasting for Buffalo Cauliflower.

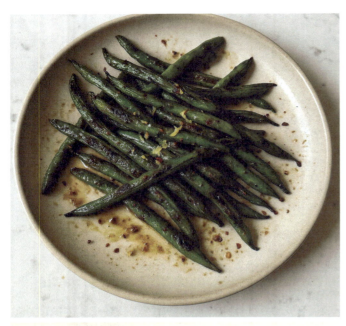

Blistered Green Beans

Servings	Prep Time	Cook time	PROTEIN	PHOSPHORUS	SODIUM	POTASSIUM
1	5'	10'	MID	LOW	LOW	MID

INGREDIENTS
- 8 oz Fresh green beans (trimmed)
- 1.5 tbsp Vegetable oil
- 1 tbsp Unsalted butter
- ½ Lemon (zest only)
- Pinch Red pepper flakes

DIRECTIONS
1. Wash and dry green beans thoroughly.
2. Heat oil in a skillet over medium-high heat.
3. Add beans and cook undisturbed for 3 minutes to blister.
4. Toss and cook 3–4 more minutes.
5. Stir in butter and lemon zest off the heat.

Nutritional Info (per serving)
Calories: 165kcal | Protein: 2g | Potassium: 260mg | Phosphorus: 40mg | Sodium: 6mg | Fat: 14g | Carbs: 8g | Cholesterol: 15mg | Oxalates: Moderate

Creativity TWIST:
Add 1 tablespoon of slivered almonds total for crunch without overloading phosphorus.

Sautéed Cabbage with Cider Vinegar

Servings	Prep Time	Cook time	PROTEIN	PHOSPHORUS	SODIUM	POTASSIUM
2	10'	15'	MID	MID	LOW	MID

INGREDIENTS
- 2 cups Green cabbage (shredded)
- ¼ Yellow onion (sliced thin)
- 2.5 tbsp Vegetable oil
- 1 tbsp Apple cider vinegar
- ½ tsp White sugar
- Black pepper

DIRECTIONS
1. Heat oil in a large skillet. Sauté onion for 5 minutes.
2. Add cabbage and cook 8–10 minutes until wilted.
3. Add vinegar and sugar; cook 1 minute to glaze.
4. Season with pepper.

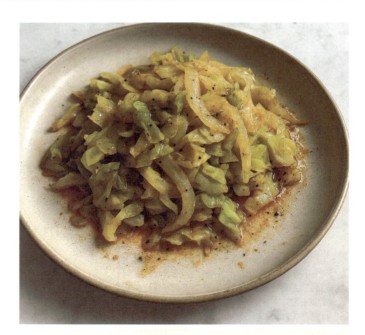

Nutritional Info (per serving)
Calories: 160kcal | Protein: 1.5g | Potassium: 180mg | Phosphorus: 30mg | Sodium: 11mg | Fat: 17g | Carbs: 8g | Cholesterol: 0mg | Oxalates: Low

Creativity TWIST:
Add a pinch of caraway seeds for a German-style flavor profile that pairs well with pork substitutes.

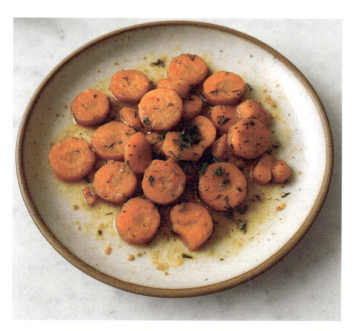

Honey-Dill Glazed Carrots

Servings	Prep Time	Cook time	PROTEIN	PHOSPHORUS	SODIUM	POTASSIUM
2	5'	15'	LOW	LOW	LOW	LOW

INGREDIENTS
- 2 large Carrots (peeled and sliced into coins)
- 2 cups Water (for boiling)
- 1.5 tbsp Unsalted butter
- 1 tbsp Honey
- 1 tbsp Fresh dill (chopped)

DIRECTIONS
1. Boil carrots in water for 10 minutes (reduces potassium/oxalates).
2. Drain well.
3. Return to pot with butter and honey. Toss over low heat to glaze.
4. Stir in fresh dill.

Nutritional Info (per serving)
Calories: 155kcal | Protein: 1g | Potassium: 220mg | Phosphorus: 30mg | Sodium: 50mg | Fat: 9g | Carbs: 18g | Cholesterol: 22mg | Oxalates: 30mg

Creativity TWIST:
Use maple syrup instead of honey and add a dash of cinnamon for an autumn version

Roasted Red Pepper & Onion Medley

Servings	Prep Time	Cook time	PROTEIN	PHOSPHORUS	SODIUM	POTASSIUM
2	10'	20'	LOW	LOW	LOW	LOW

INGREDIENTS
- 1 Red bell pepper (seeded, chunked)
- ½ large Red onion (wedged)
- 2 tbsp Olive oil
- ½ tsp Italian seasoning (salt-free)
- Black pepper

DIRECTIONS
1. Preheat oven to 400°F (200°C).
2. Toss peppers and onions with olive oil and seasoning.
3. Roast on baking sheet for 20 minutes until soft and slightly charred.

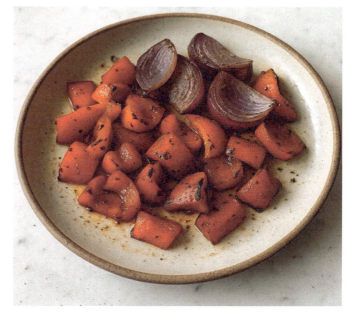

Nutritional Info (per serving)
Calories: 165kcal | Protein: 1.5g | Potassium: 210mg | Phosphorus: 30mg | Sodium: 5mg | Fat: 14g | Carbs: 9g | Cholesterol: 0mg | Oxalates: Low

Creativity TWIST:
Drizzle with a little Balsamic glaze right before serving for a sweet, acidic finish.

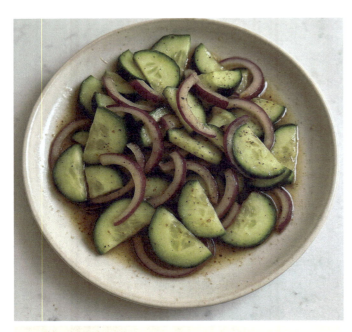

Cucumber Onion Sweet Vinaigrette

Servings	Prep Time	Cook time	PROTEIN	PHOSPHORUS	SODIUM	POTASSIUM
2	30'	0'	LOW	LOW	LOW	LOW

INGREDIENTS
- 1 large Cucumber (peeled, sliced)
- ¼ Red onion (sliced thin)
- 2 tbsp Olive oil
- ¼ cup White vinegar
- 2 tbsp White sugar
- ½ tsp Dried dill

DIRECTIONS
1. Whisk olive oil, vinegar, sugar, and dill until combined.
2. Pour over cucumbers and onions in a bowl.
3. Refrigerate 30 mins.

Nutritional Info (per serving)
Calories: 190kcal | Protein: 1g | Potassium: 160mg | Phosphorus: 25mg | Sodium: 2mg | Fat: 14g | Carbs: 16g | Cholesterol: 0mg | Oxalates: Low

Creativity TWIST:
Add a dash of celery seed (not celery salt) for an old-fashioned deli flavor.

Zucchini & Corn Sauté

Servings	Prep Time	Cook time	PROTEIN	PHOSPHORUS	SODIUM	POTASSIUM
2	5'	8'	LOW	LOW	LOW	MID

INGREDIENTS
- 1 medium Zucchini (diced)
- ½ cup Frozen corn (thawed) or Canned (rinsed)
- 2 tbsp Olive oil
- ¼ tsp Garlic powder
- Black pepper

DIRECTIONS
1. Heat oil in skillet.
2. Sauté zucchini 4 minutes.
3. Add corn and garlic powder; cook 4 more minutes.
4. Season with pepper.

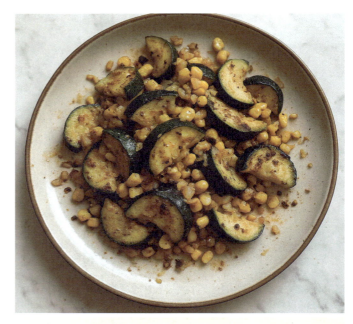

Nutritional Info (per serving)
Calories: 170kcal | Protein: 2g | Potassium: 320mg | Phosphorus: 60mg | Sodium: 10mg | Fat: 14g | Carbs: 12g | Cholesterol: 0mg | Oxalates: Moderate

Creativity TWIST:
Add fresh chopped cilantro and a squeeze of lime at the end for a taco-style side dish.

New England Light Clam Chowder

Servings	Prep Time	Cook time	PROTEIN	PHOSPHORUS	SODIUM	K POTASSIUM
2	10'	15'	MID	LOW	LOW	MID

INGREDIENTS
- 1/2 cup + 2 Tbsp (100g) canned clams, rinsed well
- 1/3 small peeled potato, diced and soaked (80g)
- 1/4 cup onion, diced (40g)
- 1 cup unsweetened almond milk (240 ml)
- 2 Tbsp extra virgin olive oil (30 ml) (pantry)
- 1 egg white (~33g)
- 1 cup water (240 ml)

DIRECTIONS
1. Sauté onion and potato in 1 Tbsp olive oil until softened.
2. Add clams, egg white, and water. Simmer for 10 min.
3. Add almond milk and remaining 1 Tbsp olive oil, heat gently.

Recommended Side Dish
Toasted Sourdough (Classic Combo)

Nutritional Info (per serving)
Calories: ~474 kcal | Protein: 14.3 g | Potassium: 420 mg | Phosphorus: 134 mg | Sodium: 232 mg | Fat: 17 g | Carbs: 12 g | Cholesterol: 30 mg | Oxalates: ~7 mg

Creativity TWIST:
Add thyme or a few drops of white wine vinegar for flavor without adding sodium.

Soft Broccoli Cheddar Whisper

Servings	Prep Time	Cook time	PROTEIN	PHOSPHORUS	SODIUM	K POTASSIUM
2	5'	15'	LOW	LOW	LOW	MID

INGREDIENTS
- 1/2 cup (45 g) broccoli florets, boiled, chopped
- 1/4 cup (30 g) peeled potato, soaked, chopped
- 1/4 cup (40 g) onion, diced
- 1/2 cup (120 ml) rice milk (pantry)
- 55 g mild cheddar cheese (garnish)
- 1.5 Tbsp (21 g) olive oil (pantry)

DIRECTIONS
1. Sauté onion, potato, and broccoli in 1.5 Tbsp olive oil until softened.
2. Add water to cover veggies and simmer until soft.
3. Blend cooked vegetables with rice milk until smooth.
4. Garnish with mild cheddar cheese.

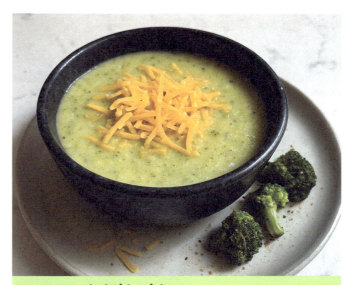

Recommended Side Dish
Roasted Red Pepper & Onion (Adds bite)

Nutritional Info (per serving)
Calories: 520 kcal | Protein: 16 g | Potassium: 309 mg | Phosphorus: 280 mg | Sodium: 280 mg | Fat: 24 g | Carbs: 16 g | Cholesterol: 10 mg | Oxalates: 4 mg

Creativity TWIST:
Use garlic powder or nutmeg to lift the flavor. Or use lactose free cheese instead of cheddar.

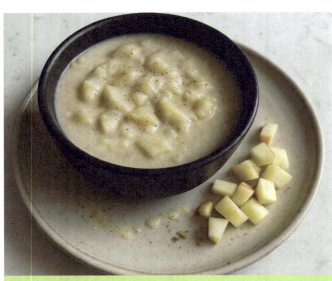

Recommended Side Dish
Blistered Green Beans (Green veg needed)

Nutritional Info (per serving)
Calories: ~460 kcal | Protein: ~15 g | Potassium: ~410 mg | Phosphorus: ~70 mg | Sodium: ~175 mg | Fat: ~24 g | Carbs: ~40 g | Cholesterol: 0 mg | Oxalates: ~13 mg

Rustic Creamy Potato Bowl

Servings	Prep Time	Cook time	PROTEIN	PHOSPHORUS	SODIUM	POTASSIUM
2	5'	15'	MID	LOW	LOW	MID

INGREDIENTS
- **240 g peeled potato, soaked and diced (~1 medium small potato)**
- **1/4 cup (25 g) leeks or onion, diced**
- **1/4 cup (30 g) peeled apple, diced**
- **1 cup (240 ml) water (pantry)**
- **1/2 cup (120 ml) unsweetened rice milk**
- **6 egg whites (~180 g)**
- **3.5 Tbsp olive oil (pantry)**

DIRECTIONS
1. Sauté leeks and apple in 2 Tbsp olive oil until softened.
2. Add potato and water, simmer until potato is soft (about 15 minutes).
3. Blend cooked mixture smooth with rice milk and egg whites.
4. Stir in remaining 1.5 Tbsp olive oil for richness and creaminess.

Creativity TWIST:
Add dill or chives for an herbal edge. For a smoky twist, try adding a pinch of smoked paprika.

Gentle Beef Stew Sipper

Servings	Prep Time	Cook time	PROTEIN	PHOSPHORUS	SODIUM	POTASSIUM
2	10'	20'	MID	MID	LOW	MID

INGREDIENTS
- **4 oz (113 g) ground beef (90% lean)**
- **2 Tbsp (15 g) diced peeled potato, soaked**
- **1/4 cup (30 g) carrots, chopped**
- **1/8 cup (15 g) celery, chopped**
- **3 Tbsp (45 ml) extra virgin olive oil (pantry)**
- **1.5 cups (360 ml) water**
- **Pepper and herbs (pantry)**

DIRECTIONS
1. Brown beef in 3 Tbsp EVOO with vegetables.
2. Add water and simmer for 15 min.
3. Skim any fat off. Season lightly with herbs.

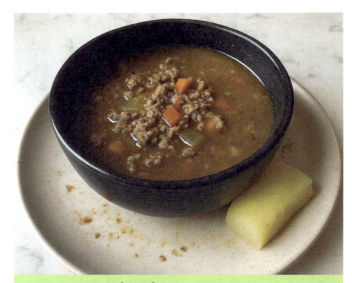

Recommended Side Dish
Lemon-Parsley White Rice (Over rice)

Nutritional Info (per serving)
Calories: 491 kcal | Protein: 13 g | Potassium: 379 mg | Phosphorus: 128 mg | Sodium: 66 mg | Fat: 32 g | Carbs: 7 g | Cholesterol: 37 mg | Oxalates: 6 mg

Creativity TWIST:
Try adding rosemary or smoked paprika for depth. Substitute celery with fennel for a milder flavor

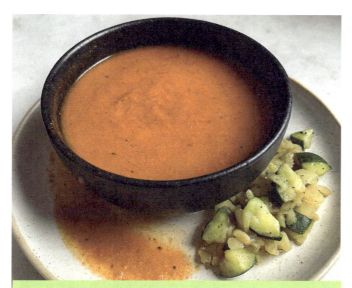

Recommended Side Dish
Toasted Sourdough (Classic Combo)

Nutritional Info (per serving)
Calories: 506 kcal | Protein: 14.7 g | Potassium: 535 mg
| Phosphorus: 59.5 mg | Sodium: 208 mg | Fat: 42.7 g |
Carbs: 16 g | Cholesterol: 0 mg | Oxalates: ~4.5 mg

Creamy Tomato Classic

Servings	Prep Time	Cook time	PROTEIN	PHOSPHORUS	SODIUM	K POTASSIUM
2	5'	15'	LOW	LOW	LOW	MID

INGREDIENTS
- 1 cup (240 g) no-salt-added crushed tomatoes (pantry)
- 1/2 cup (60 g) peeled, diced zucchini
- 1/4 cup (40 g) onion, diced
- 1/3 cup (80 ml) unsweetened rice milk
- 6 Tbsp (90 ml) extra virgin olive oil (EVOO) (pantry)
- 7 large egg whites

DIRECTIONS
1. Sauté onion and zucchini in olive oil until onion is translucent.
2. Add tomato and water. Simmer for 10 minutes.
3. Stir in rice milk and egg whites. Blend for smoothness if desired.

Creativity TWIST:
For variation, swap zucchini with yellow squash or add roasted red peppers for sweetness.

Velvety Cream of Mushroom & Chicken

Servings	Prep Time	Cook time	PROTEIN	PHOSPHORUS	SODIUM	K POTASSIUM
2	10'	15'	MID	MID	LOW	LOW

INGREDIENTS
- 1/2 cup (35 g) mushrooms, sliced
- 1/4 cup (40 g) onion, diced
- 3 oz (85 g) cooked, diced chicken breast (skinless)
- 3/4 cup (180 ml) rice milk
- 1 cup (240 ml) water
- 5 1/2 Tbsp (82.5 ml) extra virgin olive oil (pantry)

DIRECTIONS
1. Heat 5 1/2 Tbsp EVOO in a pan over medium heat.
2. Sauté mushrooms and onions until soft and fragrant.
3. Add cooked diced chicken and water; simmer gently to warm through (~5 minutes).
4. Stir in rice milk and cook for an additional 2 minutes, stirring occasionally.
5. Serve warm.

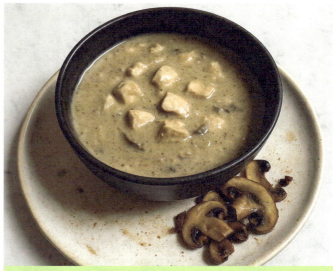

Recommended Side Dish
Toasted Sourdough

Nutritional Info (per serving)
Calories: 458 kcal | Protein: 13.8 g | Potassium: 274 mg
| Phosphorus: 136 mg | Sodium: 48 mg | Fat: 39.4 g |
Carbs: 11.6 g | Cholesterol: 35 mg | Oxalates: 3 mg

Creativity TWIST:
Try swapping mushrooms for cremini or shiitake for a deeper umami flavor.

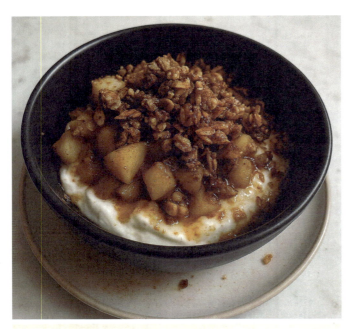

Colonial Apple Crisp Parfait

Servings	Prep Time	Cook time	PROTEIN	PHOSPHORUS	SODIUM	POTASSIUM
1	10'	12'	LOW	LOW	LOW	MID

INGREDIENTS
- ⅓ medium apple, peeled & diced (~53 g)
- ¼ cup rolled oats (21 g)
- ½ cup plain non-fat Greek yogurt (113 g)
- 1 Tbsp honey (or maple syrup) (21 g)
- 1 tsp olive oil (4.5 g) (pantry)
- ¼ tsp ground cinnamon (pantry)

DIRECTIONS
1. Warm a small skillet over medium heat. Add olive oil, oats, and cinnamon. Toast 3-4 min until fragrant.
2. Stir in diced apple; cook 5-6 min, just until soft. Drizzle half the honey; remove from heat.
3. Layer yogurt and warm apple oat mix in a parfait glass. Then add remaining honey
4. Serve warm or chilled.

Nutritional Info (per serving)
Calories: 281 kcal | Protein: 14.5 g | Potassium: 325 mg | Phosphorus: 167 mg | Sodium: 50 mg | Fat: 6.1 g | Carbs: 44 g | Cholesterol: 3 mg | Oxalates: [N/A]

Creativity TWIST:
Try swapping the apple for a pear or fresh berries to reduce potassium even more.

Broadway Cheesecake Clouds

Servings	Prep Time	Cook time	PROTEIN	PHOSPHORUS	SODIUM	POTASSIUM
1	18'	0'	LOW	LOW	LOW	LOW

INGREDIENTS
- ⅓ cup plain Greek yogurt (80 g)
- 3 oz light cream cheese, softened (85 g)
- 2 Tbsp graham-cracker crumbs (14 g)
- 1 ½ Tbsp honey (21 g) (Pantry)
- ¼ tsp pure vanilla extract

DIRECTIONS
1. Beat cream cheese, yogurt, honey, and vanilla until fluffy with a hand mixer.
2. Spoon into a ramekin; then sprinkle with graham cracker crumbs.
3. Chill 10 minutes for flavors to mix. Enjoy

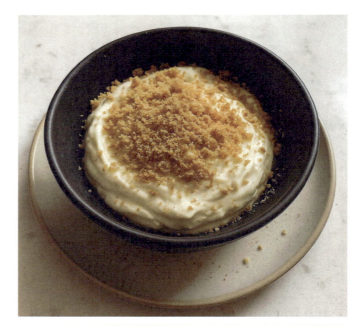

Nutritional Info (per serving)
Calories: 322 kcal | Protein: 17.7 g | Potassium: 230 mg | Phosphorus: 211 mg | Sodium: 251 mg | Fat: 15.2 g | Carbs: 34.5 g | Cholesterol: 45 mg | Oxalates: N/A

Creativity TWIST:
Top with two sliced strawberries in New York style.

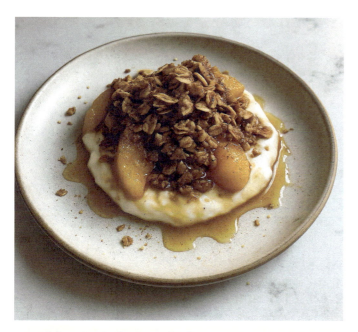

Savannah Peach Cobbler Cups

Servings	Prep Time	Cook time	PROTEIN	PHOSPHORUS	SODIUM	POTASSIUM
1	7'	10'	LOW	LOW	LOW	LOW

INGREDIENTS
- ½ cup (120 g) sliced no-sugar-added canned peaches, drained
- ¼ cup (21 g) rolled oats
- ½ cup (120 g) plain Greek yogurt
- 1 Tbsp (21 g) honey
- 1 tsp (4.5 g) olive oil (pantry) + dash cinnamon (pantry)

DIRECTIONS
1. Toast oats in olive oil with cinnamon for 3 minutes.
2. Add peaches and sauté until warmed and syrupy, about 5-6 minutes.
3. Spoon yogurt into a cu p. Crown with warm peach-oat topping and drizzle with honey

Nutritional Info (per serving)
Calories: 305 kcal | Protein: 13.5 g | Potassium: 345 mg | Phosphorus: 200 mg | Sodium: 56 mg | Fat: 6.5 g | Carbs: 49.3 g | Cholesterol: 5 mg | Oxalates: N/A

Creativity TWIST:
Sprinkle a pinch of ground cardamom for Southern meets Indian flair.

Route 66 Strawberry Shortcake Layers

Servings	Prep Time	Cook time	PROTEIN	PHOSPHORUS	SODIUM	POTASSIUM
1	6'	0'	MID	MID	LOW	MID

INGREDIENTS
- ¾ cup (184 g) plain Greek yogurt
- 1 slice angel-food cake (≈ 40 g), cubed
- ⅓ cup (50 g) sliced strawberries
- 1 Tbsp (21 g) honey
- ¼ tsp vanilla (pantry)

DIRECTIONS
1. Whisk honey, vanilla, and Greek yogurt together.
2. Layer half the cake cubes, yogurt mixture, and strawberries in a glass; repeat the layers.
3. Serve immediately. This is a soft, easy-to-chew treat.

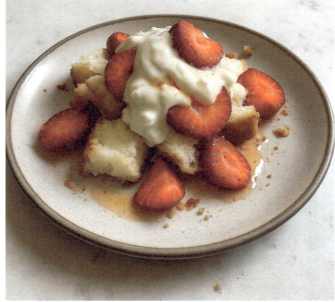

Nutritional Info (per serving)
Calories: 308 kcal | Protein: 22 g | Potassium: 503 mg | Phosphorus: 280 mg | Sodium: 232 mg | Fat: 1 g | Carbs: 53 g | Cholesterol: 10 mg | Oxalates: N/A

Creativity TWIST:
Use diced ripe peaches in summer for a Route 66 "roadside" twist.

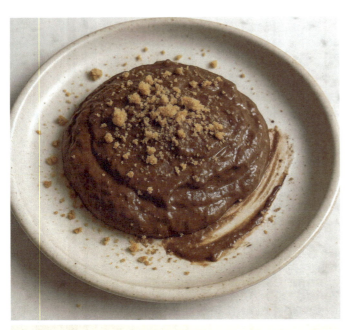

Golden Gate Chocolate Satin Pudding

Servings	Prep Time	Cook time	PROTEIN	PHOSPHORUS	SODIUM	POTASSIUM
1	5'	0'	LOW	LOW	LOW	LOW

INGREDIENTS
- ¾ cup (170g) low-fat plain Greek yogurt
- 2 Tbsp (10g) unsweetened cocoa powder
- ⅓ small ripe banana, mashed (approx 40g)
- 1 Tbsp (21g) honey
- ¼ tsp (1.25g) vanilla extract (pantry)

DIRECTIONS
1. Blend all ingredients until silky smooth.
2. Chill 10 minutes for flavors to meld.
3. Enjoy for a mousse-like texture..

Nutritional Info (per serving)
Calories: 267 kcal | Protein: 20.4 g | Potassium: 425 mg | Phosphorus: 222 mg | Sodium: 46 mg | Fat: 4.5 g | Carbs: 35.1 g | Cholesterol: 10 mg | Oxalates: Trace

Creativity TWIST:
Dust with a pinch of instant espresso powder for Mocha Bay vibes.

Homestead Cinnamon-Oat Cookie Bites

Servings	Prep Time	Cook time	PROTEIN	PHOSPHORUS	SODIUM	POTASSIUM
2	8'	12'	LOW	LOW	LOW	LOW

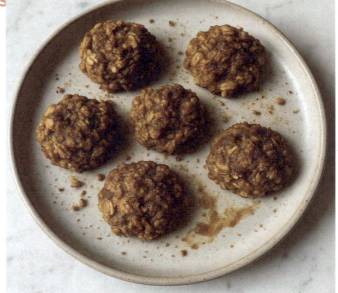

INGREDIENTS
- ½ cup rolled oats (40 g)
- ½ cup unsweetened applesauce (122 g)
- ¼ cup plain Greek yogurt, nonfat (60 g)
- 2 Tbsp honey (42 g) (Pantry)
- ½ tsp ground cinnamon (Pantry)

DIRECTIONS
1. Preheat oven to 350 °F (175 °C).
2. Stir all ingredients together until a thick dough forms.
3. Drop 6 rounded spoonfuls onto a parchment-lined baking sheet.
4. Bake for 12 minutes until done. Cool before serving.

Nutritional Info (per serving)
Calories: 184 kcal | Protein: 5.85 g | Potassium: 180.5 mg | Phosphorus: 129.5 mg | Sodium: 18.5 mg | Fat: 1.5 g | Carbs: 39.75 g | Cholesterol: 2.5 mg | Oxalates: N/A

Creativity TWIST:
Add a teaspoon of grated orange zest for a farmhouse "snickerdoodle" flair.

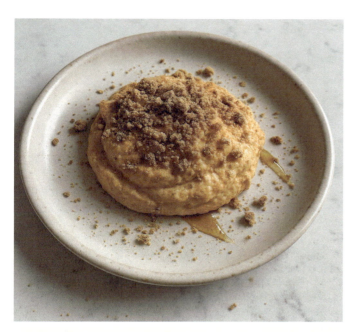

Harvest Moon Pumpkin Mousse

Servings	Prep Time	Cook time	PROTEIN	PHOSPHORUS	SODIUM	POTASSIUM
1	7'	10'	LOW	LOW	LOW	MID

INGREDIENTS
- 2 Tbsp canned pumpkin purée
- ½ cup plain Greek yogurt (~120 g)
- 1 pasteurized egg white, whipped to soft peaks (~33 g)
- 2 Tbsp graham cracker crumbs(~14 g)
- 1 Tbsp honey (pantry) (~21 g)

DIRECTIONS
1. Blend pumpkin purée, Greek yogurt, and honey until smooth.
2. Gently fold in whipped egg white to lighten.
3. Spoon mixture into a glass; top with graham cracker crumbs. Serve chilled.

Nutritional Info (per serving)
Calories: ~215 kcal | Protein: ~19 g | Potassium: ~330 mg | Phosphorus: ~190 mg | Sodium: ~150 mg | Fat: ~1.5 g | Carbs: ~29 g | Cholesterol: ~5 mg | Oxalates: N/A

Creativity TWIST:
Dust with pumpkin pie spice or use crushed ginger snap cookies instead of graham crackers.

Key Largo Lime Cream Cups

Servings	Prep Time	Cook time	PROTEIN	PHOSPHORUS	SODIUM	POTASSIUM
1	7'	0'	LOW	LOW	LOW	LOW

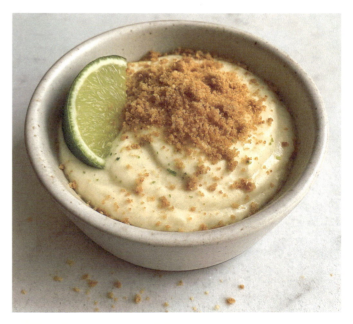

INGREDIENTS
- ¾ cup (170 g) plain Greek yogurt
- 1.25 oz (35 g) light cream cheese, softened
- ½ fresh lime, juice and zest
- 1 Tbsp (21 g) honey (pantry)
- 1 Tbsp (7 g) graham cracker crumbs

DIRECTIONS
- Whip yogurt, cream cheese, honey, and lime juice/zest until creamy.
- Spoon into a ramekin; sprinkle crumbs on to p.
- Chill 5-10 minutes for a cool Key West bite.

Nutritional Info (per serving)
Calories: 257 kcal | Protein: 19.8 g | Potassium: 316 mg | Phosphorus: 236 mg | Sodium: 221 mg | Fat: 6.5 g | Carbs: 31.7 g | Cholesterol: 24 mg | Oxalates: N/A

Creativity TWIST:
For a "sunset" cup, swirl in 1 tsp strawberry purée before chilling.

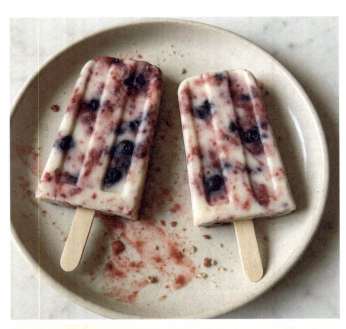

Stars & Stripes Berry Yogurt Pops

Servings	Prep Time	Cook time	PROTEIN	PHOSPHORUS	SODIUM	POTASSIUM
2	5'	4 hrs Freeze	LOW	LOW	LOW	LOW

INGREDIENTS
- ½ cup (72 g) sliced strawberries
- ½ cup (74 g) blueberries
- 1 cup (245 g) plain nonfat Greek yogurt
- 2 Tbsp (42 g) honey (pantry)

DIRECTIONS
1. Blitz berries and honey into a chunky purée.
2. Marble the purée through the yogurt.
3. Pour into two ice-pop molds; freeze for at least 4 hours.
4. Then enjoy.

Nutritional Info (per serving)
Calories: 162 kcal | Protein: 12 g | Potassium: 214 mg | Phosphorus: 129 mg | Sodium: 32 mg | Fat: 0.4 g | Carbs: 30 g | Cholesterol: 5 mg | Oxalates: N/A

Creativity TWIST:
Layer red (strawberry), white (plain yogurt), and blue (blueberry) for a patriotic look.

Boardwalk Chocolate-Chip "Nice" Cream

Servings	Prep Time	Cook time	PROTEIN	PHOSPHORUS	SODIUM	POTASSIUM
1	5'	30'	LOW	LOW	LOW	LOW

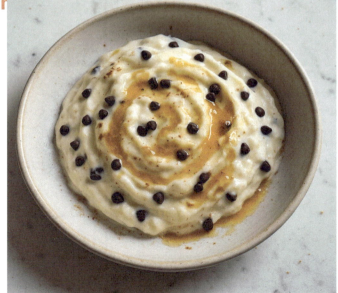

INGREDIENTS
- ¼ frozen ripe banana, sliced (about 30 g)
- ½ cup plain Greek yogurt (120 ml)
- 1 Tbsp mini dark chocolate chips (15 ml / ~15 g)
- 1 ½ Tbsp honey (22 ml) (Pantry)
- ¼ tsp vanilla extract (1.25 ml) (Pantry)

DIRECTIONS
1. In a blender, combine banana, yogurt, honey, and vanilla extract until creamy.
2. Pour mixture into a bowl. Fold in chocolate chips.
3. Enjoy this dessert soft-serve style or freeze for 30 minutes for a firmer, scoopable texture.

Nutritional Info (per serving)
Calories: 271 kcal | Protein: 12.3 g | Potassium: 391 mg | Phosphorus: 120 mg | Sodium: 31.5 mg | Fat: 4.4 g | Carbs: 46.5 g | Cholesterol: 7 mg | Oxalates: N/A

Creativity TWIST:
Add a cinnamon sprinkle for a Jersey Shore churro vibe—without extra phosphorus.

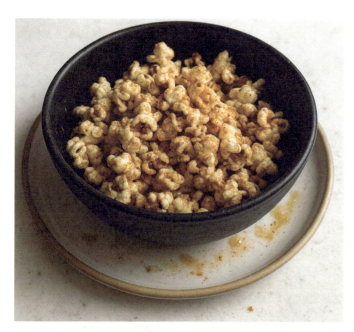

Liberty Honey-Cinnamon Popcorn

Servings	Prep Time	Cook Time	PROTEIN	PHOSPHORUS	SODIUM	POTASSIUM
1	2'	3'	LOW	LOW	LOW	LOW

INGREDIENTS
- **3 cups air-popped popcorn, unsalted (about 24 g)**
- **1 Tbsp honey (21 g) (Pantry)**
- **¼ tsp ground cinnamon (0.5 g) (Pantry)**
- **½ tsp olive oil (2.5 ml) (Pantry)**

DIRECTIONS
1. **Pop kernels in an air popper or covered saucepan.**
2. **While hot, drizzle with olive oil and warmed honey.**
3. **Add ground cinnamon. Toss to coat evenly. Serve warm.**

Nutritional Info (per serving)
Calories: 184 kcal | Protein: 3 g | Potassium: 80 mg | Phosphorus: 90 mg | Sodium: 10 mg | Fat: 4 g | Carbs: 40 g | Cholesterol: 0 mg

Creativity TWIST:
Smoked paprika will give this recipe a sweet savory kettle corn vibe.

Harvest Apple-PB Rice Cakes

Servings	Prep Time	Cook Time	PROTEIN	PHOSPHORUS	SODIUM	POTASSIUM
1	4'	3'	LOW	LOW	LOW	LOW

INGREDIENTS
- **2 mini unsalted rice cakes (18 g)**
- **2 Tbsp natural peanut butter (32 g)**
- **6 thin slices apple (½ small apple, 40 g)**
- **1 tsp honey (7 g) (Pantry)**

DIRECTIONS
1. **Spread peanut butter evenly on the rice cakes.**
2. **Top with thin apple slices.**
3. **Drizzle honey over the apple slices.**

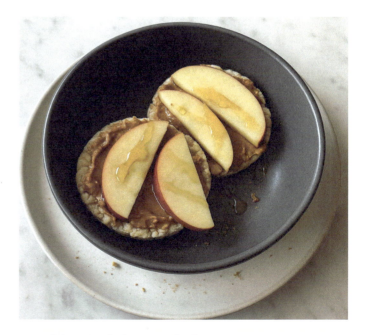

Nutritional Info (per serving)
Calories: 300 kcal | Protein: 9.5 g | Potassium: 312 mg | Phosphorus: 175 mg | Sodium: 1.4 mg | Fat: 16.5 g | Carbs: 32.2 g | Cholesterol: 0 mg

Creativity TWIST:
Dust with apple pie spice or try walnut butter instead.

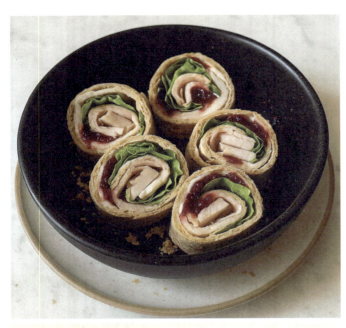

Route 66 Turkey-Cranberry Roll-Up

Servings	Prep Time	Cook time	PROTEIN	PHOSPHORUS	SODIUM	POTASSIUM
1	5'	3'	LOW	LOW	MID	MID

INGREDIENTS
- 1 small (30 g) low-sodium whole-wheat tortilla
- 2 oz (56 g) sliced low-sodium turkey breast
- 1 TBL (14 g) reduced-fat cream cheese
- 1 TBL (15 g) reduced-sugar cranberry sauce
- 3 leaves (15 g) butter lettuce (soft)

DIRECTIONS
1. Spread cream cheese evenly over the tortilla.
2. Layer turkey slices, butter lettuce, and cranberry sauce on to p.
3. Roll tightly and slice into bite-sized pinwheels.

Nutritional Info (per serving)
Calories: 217 kcal | Protein: 16.2 g | Potassium: 345 mg | Phosphorus: 243 mg | Sodium: 385 mg | Fat: 7 g | Carbs: 22.4 g | Cholesterol: 40 mg | Oxalates: [N/A]

CREATIVITY TWIST:
Warm briefly in a dry skillet for a "melted" version.

Bayou Deviled Egg Halves

Servings	Prep Time	Cook time	PROTEIN	PHOSPHORUS	SODIUM	POTASSIUM
1	5'	10'	LOW	LOW	LOW	LOW

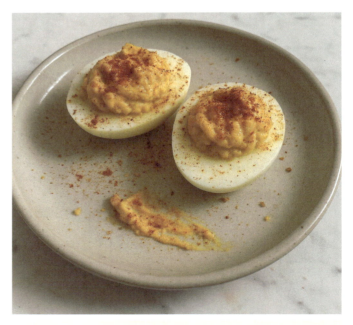

INGREDIENTS
- 1 large egg
- 1 tsp low-sodium mayonnaise (5 g)
- ¼ tsp yellow mustard (1.2 g)
- Pinch paprika (0.2 g) (pantry)

DIRECTIONS
1. Hard-boil the egg. Cool, peel, and halve the egg.
2. Mash the yolk. Add mayonnaise and mustard; mix well.
3. Pipe the mixture back into the egg white halves.
4. Dust with paprika. Serve.

Nutritional Info (per serving)
Calories: 106 kcal | Protein: 6.45 g | Potassium: 87 mg | Phosphorus: 106 mg | Sodium: 151 mg | Fat: 8.4 g | Carbs: 0.9 g | Cholesterol: 191 mg | Oxalates: negligible

Creativity TWIST:
Add a few drops of hot sauce or minced chives for flavor.

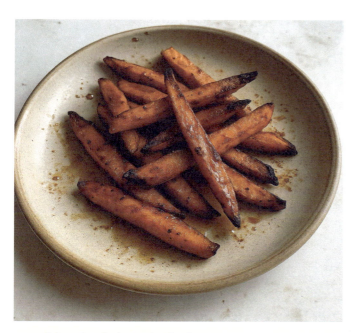

Nutritional Info (per serving)

Calories: 377 kcal | Protein: 2.25 g | Potassium: 502 mg |
Phosphorus: 32 mg | Sodium: 58 mg | Fat: 27.2 g | Carbs:
32.8 g | Cholesterol: 0 mg | Oxalates: N/A

Sunset Sweet-Potato Fries

Servings	Prep Time	Cook time	PROTEIN	PHOSPHORUS	SODIUM	POTASSIUM
1	5'	20'	LOW	LOW	MID	MID

INGREDIENTS

- 1 small sweet potato, peeled, cut into thin wedges (about 130 g)
- 2 Tbsp (30 ml) olive oil (pantry)
- ¼ tsp (0.75 g) garlic powder (pantry)
- ¼ tsp (0.5 g) smoked paprika (pantry)
- 1 tsp (7 g) honey (optional glaze)

DIRECTIONS

1. Toss wedges with olive oil, garlic powder, and smoked paprika in a plastic bag.
2. Bake at 425 °F / 220 °C for 15–20 minutes on a sheet pan, turning once halfway through.
3. Drizzle honey over fries just before serving (optional).

Creativity TWIST:
Try this recipe with cinnamon instead of smoked paprika for a sweeter, warmer twist.

Windy City Mozzarella Melts

Servings	Prep Time	Cook time	PROTEIN	PHOSPHORUS	SODIUM	POTASSIUM
1	4'	2'	LOW	LOW	LOW	LOW

INGREDIENTS

- 4 unsalted mini rice cakes
- 1 oz (28 g) part-skim mozzarella, shredded
- 2 thin seeded tomato slices (~20 g)
- 3 fresh basil leaves, torn (~1 g)
- ½ tsp (2.5 ml) olive oil

DIRECTIONS

1. Arrange rice cakes on a microwave-safe plate.
2. Top rice cakes with tomato slices and shredded mozzarella.
3. Microwave for 20–40 seconds until the cheese melts.
4. Drizzle olive oil on top and sprinkle torn basil leaves.

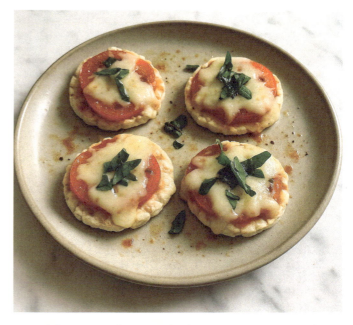

Nutritional Info (per serving)

Calories: 202 kcal | Protein: 9.0 g | Potassium: 110 mg
| Phosphorus: 185 mg | Sodium: 176 mg | Fat: 7.6 g |
Carbs: 26 g | Cholesterol: 22 mg | Oxalates: N/A

Creativity TWIST:
Use smoked mozzarella for a pizza or bagel flavor twist.

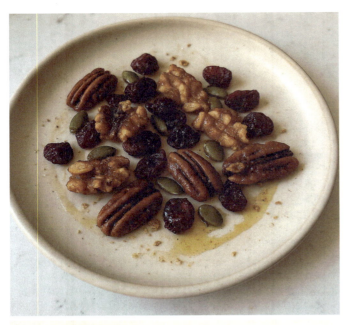

Desert Trail Nut Bowl

Servings	Prep Time	Cook time	PROTEIN	PHOSPHORUS	SODIUM	POTASSIUM
2	2'	0'	LOW	MID	LOW	LOW

INGREDIENTS
- 1 Tbsp (7.5 g) unsalted pecan halves
- 1 Tbsp (7.5 g) unsalted walnut pieces
- 1 Tbsp (9 g) dried cranberries
- 1 tsp (2.7 g) unsalted pumpkin seeds
- 1 tsp (7 g) honey (pantry)

DIRECTIONS
1. Toss all ingredients together.
2. Enjoy a handful of the mix.

Nutritional Info (per serving)
Calories: 168 kcal | Protein: 2.6 g | Potassium: 130 mg |
Phosphorus: 104 mg | Sodium: 3 mg | Fat: 11.6 g | Carbs:
16.6 g | Cholesterol: 0 mg | Oxalates: 5mg

Creativity TWIST:
Lightly toast nuts with a pinch of cinnamon for extra aroma.

Coney Island Soft-Pretzel Bites

Servings	Prep Time	Cook time	PROTEIN	PHOSPHORUS	SODIUM	POTASSIUM
1	8'	12'	LOW	LOW	MID	LOW

INGREDIENTS
- 3 oz low-sodium refrigerated pizza dough (85 g)
- 2 cups water (480 ml) (pantry)
- 1 Tbsp baking soda (15 g) (pantry)
- ½ tsp olive oil (2.5 ml) (pantry)
- ⅛ tsp coarse salt substitute (optional) (pantry)
- 1 tsp yellow mustard (5 ml)

DIRECTIONS
1. Roll dough into a ½-inch (1.3 cm) rope and cut into 1-inch (2.5 cm) pieces.
2. Boil water with baking soda; cook dough pieces for 30 seconds, then drain.
3. Place on parchment-lined pan, brush with olive oil, and sprinkle with optional salt substitute.
4. Bake at 425°F (220°C) for 10–12 minutes until golden brown.
5. Serve with yellow mustard.

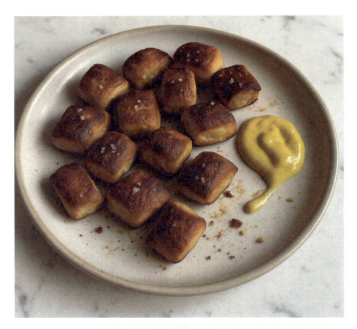

Nutritional Info (per serving)
Calories: 255 kcal | Protein: 7 g | Potassium: 110 mg |
Phosphorus: 80 mg | Sodium: 320 mg | Fat: 6 g | Carbs:
42 g | Cholesterol: 0 mg | Oxalates: N/A

Creativity TWIST:
Dust pretzel bites with cinnamon and honey instead of mustard for a sweet fair-style snack

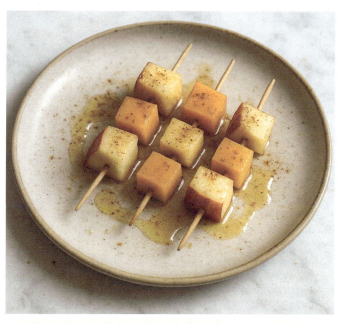

Alpine Apple-Cheddar Skewers

Servings	Prep Time	Cook time	PROTEIN	PHOSPHORUS	SODIUM	POTASSIUM
1	3'	0'	LOW	LOW	LOW	LOW

INGREDIENTS
- ½ small sweet apple, cubed (approx. 75g)
- 1 oz low-sodium cheddar, cubed (28 g)
- 1 tsp honey (7 g) (pantry)
- ⅛ tsp ground nutmeg (0.25 g) (pantry)
- 3 cocktail picks

DIRECTIONS
1. Thread alternating apple and cheese cubes on cocktail picks.
2. Drizzle honey over the skewers.
3. Lightly dust with ground nutmeg. Enjoy!

Nutritional Info (per serving)
Calories: 175 kcal | Protein: 7.3 g | Potassium: 124 mg | Phosphorus: 156 mg | Sodium: 142 mg | Fat: 9.7 g | Carbs: 17 g | Cholesterol: 29 mg | Oxalates: ~5 mg

Creativity TWIST:
Outstanding with mild goat cheese. Try adding thyme as well.

Hollywood Frozen Banana Pop

Servings	Prep Time	Cook time	PROTEIN	PHOSPHORUS	SODIUM	POTASSIUM
1	5'	1h	LOW	LOW	LOW	MID

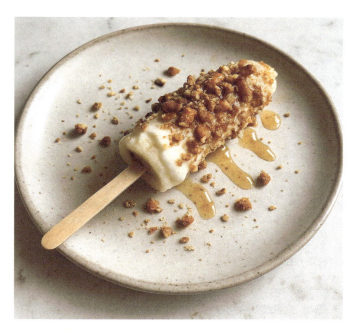

INGREDIENTS
- ½ medium banana, peeled (~58 g)
- 2 Tbsp (30 g) low-fat vanilla Greek yogurt
- 1 Tbsp (7 g) crushed unsalted pretzels
- 1 tsp (7 g) honey (pantry)
- 1 wooden stick

DIRECTIONS
1. Insert wooden stick into banana half; coat evenly with yogurt.
2. Roll coated banana in crushed pretzels; drizzle honey on to p.
3. Freeze on a plate for at least 1 hour until firm.

Nutritional Info (per serving)
Calories: 117 kcal | Protein: 4.2 g | Potassium: 258 mg | Phosphorus: 59 mg | Sodium: 12 mg | Fat: 0.5 g | Carbs: 26 g | Cholesterol: 1.5 mg | Oxalates: N/A

Creativity TWIST:
Use diced strawberries instead of pretzels for a gluten-free and lower sodium po p.

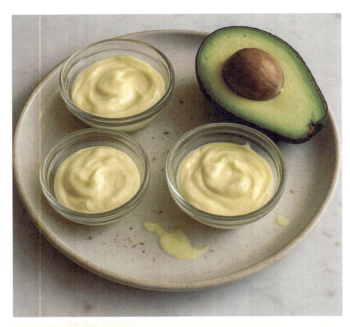

Cabo Avocado-Oil Mayo

Servings	Prep Time	Cook time	PROTEIN	PHOSPHORUS	SODIUM	POTASSIUM
1	3'	0'	LOW	LOW	LOW	LOW

INGREDIENTS
- 1 cup (240 ml) cold-pressed avocado oil
- 2 large egg yolks (about 34 g)
- 1 TBL (15 ml) fresh lemon juice
- 1 tsp (5 ml) white vinegar, optional for extra tang
- ¼ tsp salt-free herbal seasoning

DIRECTIONS
1. Place egg yolks and lemon juice in a narrow jar just wide enough for an immersion blender.
2. Blend 5 seconds to combine, then—with the blender running—slowly drizzle in the avocado oil until thick and creamy (about 60 seconds).
3. Finish with vinegar and seasoning; pulse to mix. Cover and refrigerate up to 7 days.

Nutritional Info (per serving)
Calories 102 kcal | Protein 0.14 g | Potassium 13 mg | Phosphorus 10 mg | Sodium 5 mg | Fat 11 g | Carbs 0 g | Cholesterol 9 mg | Oxalates 0 mg

Creativity TWIST:
Swap half the avocado oil for cold-pressed walnut oil for a subtle nutty note

De Baneh Balsamic Vinaigrette

Servings	Prep Time	Cook time	PROTEIN	PHOSPHORUS	SODIUM	POTASSIUM
16 Tbsp	5'	0'	LOW	LOW	LOW	MID

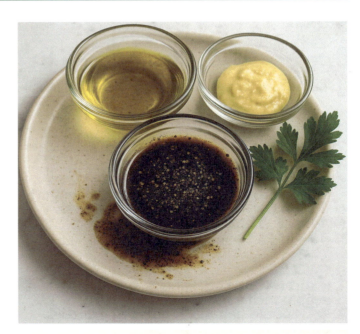

INGREDIENTS
- ¾ cup (180 ml) extra-virgin olive oil (pantry)
- ¼ cup (60 ml) aged balsamic vinegar
- 1 tsp (5 ml) Dijon-style mustard (no added salt)
- 1 tsp (2 g) fresh-ground black pepper (pantry)

DIRECTIONS
- In a screw-top jar, whisk mustard with balsamic vinegar.
- Add olive oil and herbs; seal and shake until emulsified.
- Store refrigerated up to 2 weeks; shake before serving.

Nutritional Info (per serving)
Calories 49 kcal | Protein 0 g | Potassium 6 mg | Phosphorus 1 mg | Sodium 9 mg | Fat 5.4 g | Carbs 0.7 g | Cholesterol 0 mg | Oxalates 1 mg

Creativity TWIST:
For a Tuscan riff, replace half the balsamic with red-wine vinegar and add a crushed basil leaf.

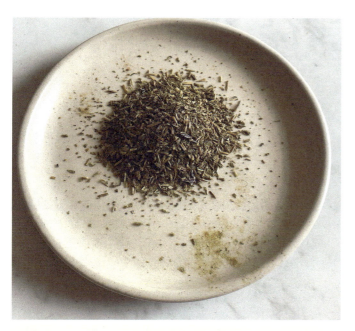

Lavender Fields Herbs de Provence

Servings	Prep Time	Cook time	PROTEIN	PHOSPHORUS	SODIUM	POTASSIUM
12 tsp	3'	0'	LOW	MID	LOW	LOW

INGREDIENTS
- 1 tsp (2 g) dried thyme
- 1 tsp (2 g) dried rosemary, crumbled
- 1 tsp (2 g) dried marjoram
- 1 tsp (2 g) dried savory or oregano
- ½ tsp (1 g) culinary lavender buds, crushed

DIRECTIONS
1. Combine all herbs; store in an airtight jar away from light up to 6 months.
2. Use ½ tsp per serving to season poultry, vegetables, or vinaigrettes.

Nutritional Info (per serving)
Calories 1 kcal | Protein 0.06 g | Potassium 10 mg | Phosphorus 2 mg | Sodium 1 mg | Fat 0.04 g | Carbs 0.2 g | Cholesterol 0 mg | Oxalates 1 mg

Creativity TWIST:
Add a pinch of dried orange zest for Mediterranean sunshine in rubs and stews.

Gentle Phos.-Free Baking Powder

Servings	Prep Time	Cook time	PROTEIN	PHOSPHORUS	SODIUM	POTASSIUM
1	8'	12'	LOW	LOW	MID	LOW

For lower sodium, substitute half the baking soda with potassium bicarbonate only if your care team approves additional potassium;

INGREDIENTS
- 6 tsp (30 g) cream of tartar
- 3 tsp (15 g) low-sodium baking soda (pantry)
- 3 tsp (15 g) non-GMO cornstarch

DIRECTIONS
1. Sift ingredients twice to distribute evenly.
2. Store airtight; use 1 tsp per cup (120 g) of flour in quick-bread recipes.

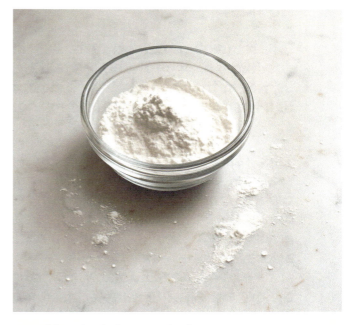

Nutritional Info (per serving)
Calories 0 kcal | Protein 0 g | Potassium 0 mg | Phosphorus 0 mg | Sodium 160 mg | Fat 0 g | Carbs 0 g | Cholesterol 0 mg | Oxalates 0 mg

Continue the Journey

You've come far. In these pages, you've learned what CKD means for your daily life and exactly how to eat better without stress or confusion. You now have simple recipes, clear shopping tips, and meal plans you can actually stick to.

Even if you just made one kidney-friendly meal, that's a big win. Every small step you take is real progress—further from dialysis, closer to more energy, better labs, and a sense of control. You don't need perfection. Just keep moving forward, one meal at a time.

But remember balancing is key so if you had a high potassium breakfast, go lighter in the next meal to balance out. Same with protein and other nutrients.

This senior-friendly book is built for real life. On tough days, when cooking feels impossible, you'll find soft, easy meals. When you're tired of complicated advice, you have clear, dietitian-approved answers. If your memory slips or you need to eat with arthritis or low energy, the simple instructions and short shopping lists will be here for you. It's your go-to guide—not just now, but for every stage ahead.

If this book helped you, consider sharing it. Grab a copy for a friend or loved one facing kidney issues. Good food and good health are always better shared.

You can write down 3 name of people you think would find this book helpful:

....

....

....

Thank you for letting me support your journey. You're stronger than you think. Keep making progress, and know I'm cheering for you every step of the way.

With love,

Marianne Greene

How helpful is this book to you?

I'd love to hear what you think.

I personally read every review, and your feedback means the world to me.It only takes 30 seconds to leave a reivew.

It truly makes a huge difference for a small author like me—and it helps other CKD warriors discover this book too.

Here's how you can leave a review for the paperback:

- **Option 1: Scan the QR code to go straight to the review page.**

- **Option 2: Go to your Amazon orders, find this book, and click "Write a product review."**
- **Option 3: Search for the book title on Amazon, scroll down to the "Customer Reviews" section, and click "Write a Review."**

Once you're there, choose a star rating, a quick story about your experience, and submit!

That's it!

Thank you so much and hope to see you in our grou p. // MARIANNE <3

JOIN OUR PRIVATE FACEBOOK GROUP!

Living with CKD can feel isolating and overwhelming, especially when it comes to diet and lifestyle changes. In this group, you're not alone. You'll gain support from a community that truly understands what you're facing, get answers to your questions, and feel empowered with encouragement and resources tailored to your needs. Just search

"KIDNEY DISEASE WARRIORS: STAGE 3 & 4 CKD DIET, RECIPES AND COMMUNITY"

The group is on Facebook—we can't wait to welcome you.

Or Scan this and request to join our group <3

If you haven't Already claimed it, Scan the code below to sign up and then download and print them:

Grab your FREE Kidney-Safe Power Tools:

◊ Get your 60 day detailed meal plan

◊ A game-changing Dining Out Cheat Sheet

◊ A CKD do-it-yourself Weekly Meal Planner to stay on track

◊ A Kidney-Friendly Grocery List for Smart Shopping

Resources

REGISTERED DIETITIANS

Matilde Ladnier RDN

Registered dietitian specializing in kidney health with over 30 years of experience. She is also a member of the National Kidney Foundation-Council of Renal Nutrition (CRN)

Email: matmirrorRD@gmail.com

Phone: +1 713.303.3052

Website:

https://matilde-ladnier.clientsecure.me/

National Kidney Foundation (NKF)

You can find registered dietitians here also. Trusted nonprofit offering clear info on CKD stages, tests, treatments, and patient mentoring programs.

www.kidney.org

MEDICAL EDUCATION

American Kidney Fund (AKF)

Provides kidney disease education, stage-by-stage guides, and financial aid info for patients.

www.kidneyfund.org

National Institute of Diabetes and Digestive and Kidney Diseases (NIDDK)

Government site with plain-language explanations of CKD causes, management, and diet tips.

niddk.nih.gov

Mayo Clinic – Chronic Kidney Disease

Comprehensive overview of CKD symptoms, diagnosis, and treatment in patient-friendly language.

www.mayoclinic.org

Kidney School

Free, interactive online education modules to learn how to manage CKD day-to-day.

kidneyschool.org

MedlinePlus – Chronic Kidney Disease

NIH consumer health site offering easy summaries, videos, and links to kidney resources.

medlineplus.gov

RENAL DIET AND MEAL PLANNING

American Kidney Fund – Kidney Kitchen

Kidney-friendly recipes, meal plans, and nutrition guides tailored for CKD diets.

kitchen.kidneyfund.org

DaVita Kidney Care – Diet & Nutrition

Hundreds of renal diet recipes, meal planning tools, and nutrition education.

davita.com/diet-nutrition

National Kidney Foundation – Nutrition Label Reading

Guidance on interpreting food labels for sodium, phosphorus, and potassium content.

www.kidney.org

Academy of Nutrition and Dietetics – Find a Renal Dietitian

Directory to locate registered dietitians specializing in kidney disease.

eatright.org/find-an-expert

Kidney Community Kitchen (Canada)

Kidney-friendly recipes and meal planning tools (metric units, international use).

kidneycommunitykitchen.ca

ONLINE SUPPORT AND COMMUNITY

NKF Kidney Community Forums (HealthUnlocked)

Active online support forums connecting CKD patients, caregivers, and experts.

healthunlocked.com/nationalkidneyfoundation

American Association of Kidney Patients (AAKP) Support Groups

Directory of in-person and virtual support groups for kidney patients and caregivers.

aak p.org/support-groups

Renal Support Network (RSN)

Patient-run nonprofit with monthly virtual support groups, podcasts, and webinars.

rsnhope.org

I Hate Dialysis Forums

Peer-to-peer online message boards for CKD patients and caregivers at all stages.

ihatedialysis.com

Facebook Support Groups

Numerous private Facebook groups offer peer support for CKD patients and families.

Search "Chronic Kidney Disease Support" on Facebook

NKF Cares Helpline

Free kidney health phone support and resource referral at 1-855-653-2273.

FINANCIAL AID AND MEDICATION HELP

American Kidney Fund Financial Assistance

Need-based grants for insurance, treatment, and related expenses for kidney patients.

kidneyfund.org/get-assistance

Medicare and SHIP

Federal and state programs helping cover CKD treatment and medication costs; call 1-800-MEDICARE or contact your local State Health Insurance Assistance Program.

Patient Access Network (PAN) Foundation

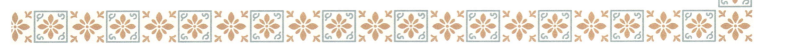

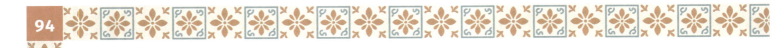

Grants for copays and treatment expenses for eligible kidney-related conditions.

panfoundation.org

HealthWell Foundation

Financial aid for medication copays and premiums for certain chronic illnesses including kidney disease.

healthwellfoundation.org

NeedyMeds

Database of prescription assistance programs to help patients afford medications.

needymeds.org

Medicine Assistance Tool (MAT)

Search engine for manufacturer prescription assistance programs by drug name.

medicineassistancetool.org

American Kidney Fund Prescription Discount Card

Free discount card to save on medications without income restrictions.

kidneyfund.org

TOOLS AND TRACKERS

DaVita Diet Helper

Interactive online meal planner that customizes renal diet meal plans and tracks nutrients.

davita.com/diet-helper

Mizu App

Mobile app for CKD patients to track symptoms, diet, and medications with reminders.

Available on iOS and Android app stores (search "Mizu CKD")

CareClinic Symptom Tracker

Mobile app for logging CKD symptoms, medications, and lifestyle habits.

careclinic.io

MediSafe

User-friendly medication reminder app with notifications and logs for patients and caregivers.

Available on iOS and Android app stores

PhosFilter App

iOS app that scans grocery barcodes to detect phosphate additives in foods.

Search "PhosFilter" in Apple App Store

Blood Pressure Monitors with App Sync

Recommended home BP monitors like Omron with apps to track and share blood pressure readings.

Printable CKD Journals

Free downloadable symptom and medication tracking sheets available on NKF and AKF websites.

Made in the USA
Monee, IL
26 November 2025

36507956R00052